Study Guide

Introduction to Clinical Pharmacology

Ninth edition

Constance G. Visovsky, PhD, RN, ACNP, FAAN
Associate Professor and Director of Diversity
College of Nursing
University of South Florida
Tampa, Florida

Cheryl H. Zambroski, PhD, RN
Associate Professor
College of Nursing
University of South Florida
Tampa, Florida

Shirley Meier Hosler, RN, BSN, MSN
Adjunct Faculty
Santa Fe Community College
Santa Fe, New Mexico

Study Guide

Introduction to Clinical Pharmacology

Ninth edition

Denise Passmore, PhD
Assistant Professor
University of South Florida College of Nursing
Tampa, Florida

ELSEVIER

ELSEVIER

3251 Riverport Lane
St. Louis, Missouri 63043

STUDY GUIDE FOR INTRODUCTION TO CLINICAL PHARMACOLOGY,   ISBN: 978-0-323-52912-9
Ninth Edition

Notices

Senior Content Strategist: Nancy O'Brien
Senior Content Development Specialist: Laura Goodrich
Publishing Service Manager: Deepthi Unni
Project Manager: Radhika Sivalingam
Cover Design: Muthukumaran Thangaraj

Printed in the United States of America

Last digit is the print number: 9   8   7   6   5   4   3   2   1

Working together
to grow libraries in
developing countries

www.elsevier.com • www.bookaid.org

To the Student

The role of the LPN/LVN is becoming increasingly important in the healthcare system, particularly as many registered nurses retire and leave the profession. More and more LPN/LVNs will move into responsible positions in a wide variety of settings—both inside and outside the United States—where this book is used. LPN/LVNs must be prepared to practice in settings with advanced technology, many other healthcare workers, and increasingly complex patients, diseases, and treatments. They must also be prepared to care for patients in areas where they may be one of the only healthcare workers; where there is no technology; and many challenging patients, diseases, and treatments.

This textbook was written in a concise and simple manner to share important information about the complex process of giving medications. It was written deliberately to provide information that LPN/LVNs must know. The Study Guide is designed to help those students who are serious about doing well on the NCLEX exams and caring well for patients. The content has been selected based on what faculty from a variety of LPN/LVN programs agree is relevant and necessary.

Learning about pharmacology and the medications to give to your patients is important. Mastering difficult concepts and tasks is often a great source of personal happiness.

STUDY HINTS FOR ALL STUDENTS

Ask Questions!

There are no stupid questions. If you do not know something or are not sure, you need to find out. Other people may be wondering the same thing but may be too shy to ask. The answer could mean life or death to your patient. That is certainly more important than feeling embarrassed about asking a question.

Chapter Objectives

At the beginning of each chapter in the textbook are objectives that you should have mastered when you finish studying that chapter. Write these objectives in your notebook, leaving a blank space after each. Fill in the answers as you find them while reading the chapter. Review to make sure your answers are correct and complete. Use these answers when you study for tests. This should also be done for separate course objectives that your instructor has listed in your class syllabus.

Evolve Website

The Evolve website to accompany the *Introduction to Clinical Pharmacology,* 8th edition textbook contains the

following resources: Animations; Answer Keys to case studies, critical thinking questions and end-of-chapter NCLEX Review Questions; Drug Dosage Calculators; an audio and English/Spanish glossary; Interactive NCLEX Review Questions; Patient Teaching Handouts; and Videoclips. Using these resources as you study can help you master the material. The Evolve website for the textbook can be found at (http://evolve.elsevier.com/Edmunds /LPN/).

Key Terms

At the beginning of each chapter in the textbook are key terms that you will encounter as you read the chapter. Text page number references are provided for easy reference and review, and the key terms are in color the first time they appear in the chapter. Phonetic pronunciations are provided for terms that you might find difficult to pronounce. The goal is to help the student reader with limited proficiency in English to develop a greater command of the pronunciation of scientific and nonscientific terminology in English. It is hoped that a more general competency in the understanding and use of medical and scientific language may result.

Key Points

Use the Key Points at the end of each chapter in the textbook to help with review for exams.

Reading Hints

When reading each chapter in the textbook, look at the subject headings to learn what each section is about. Read for the general meaning first. Then reread parts you did not understand. It may help to read those parts aloud. Carefully read the information given in each table and study each figure and its caption.

Concepts

While studying, put difficult concepts into your own words to see if you understand them. Check this understanding with another student or the instructor. Write these in your notebook.

Class Notes

When taking lecture notes in class, leave a large margin on the left side of each notebook page and write only on right-hand pages, leaving all left-hand pages blank. Look over your lecture notes soon after each class, while your memory is fresh. Fill in missing words, complete sentences and ideas, and underline key phrases, definitions, and concepts. At the top of each page, write the topic of that page. In the left margin, write the key word for that part of your notes. On the opposite left-hand page, write a summary or outline that combines material from both the textbook and the lecture. These can be your study notes for review.

Study Groups

Form a study group with other students so you can help each other. Practice speaking and reading aloud. Ask questions about material you are not sure about. Work together to find answers. Attempt to answer the textbook and syllabus objectives in your own words.

References for Improving Study Skills

Good study skills are essential for achieving your goals in nursing. Time management, efficient use of study time, and a consistent approach to studying are all beneficial. There are various study methods for reading a textbook and for taking class notes. Some methods that have proven helpful can be found in *Saunders Student Nurse Planner* by Susan deWit. This book contains helpful information on test taking and preparing for clinical experiences. It includes an example of a "time map" for planning study time and a blank form that you can use to formulate a personal time map.

ADDITIONAL STUDY HINTS FOR ESL/LEP (ENGLISH AS A SECOND-LANGUAGE/LIMITED ENGLISH PROFICIENCY) STUDENTS

First Language Buddy

ESL/LEP students should find a first-language buddy— another student who is a native speaker of English and is willing to answer questions about word meanings, pronunciations, and culture. Maybe your buddy would like to learn about your language and culture too. This could help in his or her nursing experience as well.

Vocabulary

If you find a nontechnical word you do not know (e.g., *drowsy*), try to guess its meaning from the sentence (e.g., *With electrolyte imbalance, the patient may feel fatigued and drowsy.*). If you are not sure of the meaning, or if it seems particularly important, look it up in the dictionary. (If you guessed that *drowsy* means something like sleepy, you were correct!). If there is a technical word you do not understand or remember, look for it in the index at the back of the textbook or in your medical dictionary. Write it in your notebook. Keep an alphabetical list of words you have difficulty remembering so you can look them up easily and review them before a test.

Vocabulary Notebook

Keep a small alphabetized notebook or address book in your pocket or purse. Write down new nontechnical words you read or hear along with their meanings and pronunciations. Write each word under its initial letter so you can find it easily, as in a dictionary. For words you do not know or for words that have a different meaning in nursing, write down how they sound and are used. Look up their meanings in a dictionary or ask your instructor or first-language buddy. Then write the different meanings or usages that you have found in your book, including the nursing meaning. Continue to add new words as you discover them. For example:

primary   ■ **of most importance; main:** *the primary problem or disease*
  ■ **the first one; elementary:** *primary school*
secondary   ■ **of less importance; resulting from another problem or disease:** *a secondary symptom*
  ■ **the second one:** *secondary school* **(in the United States, high school)**

Contents

1 Pharmacology and the Nursing Process in LPN Practice

TERMINOLOGY REVIEW

Match the definition with the term. Not all terms will be used.

1. _____ A health-related reason for not giving a specific drug to a patient or a group of patients.

2. _____ The act of carrying out the planned interventions.

3. _____ A drug effect that is more severe than expected and has the potential to damage tissue or cause serious health problems. It may also be called adverse effect, toxic effect, or toxicity and usually requires an intervention by the prescriber.

4. _____ The intended action of the drug, also known as a drug's beneficial outcomes.

5. _____ The process of determining the right response by looking at what happens to the patient when the nursing care plan is put into action. It is an appraisal of the treatment effectiveness.

6. _____ Information used to reliably prove an individual is the person for whom the drug treatment was intended. Identifiers may be a person's full name, the medical record identification number, birthdate, or even the telephone number.

7. _____ A name (or label) for the patient's disease or condition.

8. _____ A system to guide the nurse's work in a logical way. Consists of five major steps: (1) assessment, (2) diagnosis, (3) planning, (4) implementation, and (5) evaluation.

9. _____ A collection of information typically stored in a computer or electronic medical record.

10. _____ Reports of what the patient says he or she is feeling or thinking.

A. Adverse effect
B. Assessment
C. Contraindication
D. Database
E. Diagnosis
F. Evaluation
G. Healthcare setting
H. Implementation
I. Identifiers
J. Nine rights of drug administration
K. Nursing process
L. Objective data
M. Subjective data
N. Therapeutic effect

Match each of the following actions with the nursing process. You will use the nursing process items more than once.

11. _____ As part of the medical plan, you analyze goals and write nursing care plans.

12. _____ The healthcare team labels the patient's condition.

13. _____ You gather complete information about the patient's history of illnesses and surgeries, including any drugs the patient is currently taking.

14. _____ You give the drugs to the patient, following the plan identified by the healthcare team.

15. _____ You gather initial information that can be used as a baseline for comparison as care progresses.

16. _____ After giving the drugs, you assess the patient for any possible adverse reactions or more common side-effects.

17. _____ The identification of the patient's condition helps you identify how to teach the patient about self-care.

18. _____ You assess the patient after giving the drugs in order to determine whether the patient's condition is improving.

A. Assessment
B. Diagnosis
C. Planning
D. Implementation
E. Evaluation

Identify whether each type of information listed is (S) subjective or (O) objective data regarding the patient's health condition.

19. _____ The patient states that she is feeling nauseous.

20. _____ The patient has a temperature of 101 degrees.

21. _____ The patient's blood pressure is 140/88.

22. _____ The patient reports pain in her abdomen.

23. _____ The patient describes the feeling of pressure in her chest.

24. _____ The patient weighs 150 pounds.

25. _____ The patient has an irregular heartbeat.

List at least three follow-up questions you will need to know that relate to giving drugs.

26. _____

27. _____

28. _____

29. When taking a patient history, which of the following are important items to list that can affect the health of the patient? (Select all that apply)
☐ Prescription drugs
☐ Birth control pills
☐ Skin cream
☐ Implanted birth control devices
☐ Make-up
☐ Vitamins
☐ Marijuana
☐ Herbal therapies
☐ Tea or Coffee
☐ Cocaine
☐ Aspirin
☐ Hair gel

2

Fill in the blanks. What additional information do you need to know to manage drug administration?

30. _____ that include the name of the drug and the type of reaction the patient experienced (in other words, was it a mild or severe effect).

31. _____ that may prohibit or limit use of some drugs (such as sickle cell disease, glucose-6-phosphate dehydrogenase deficiency, history of drug addiction, or immune deficiencies)

Planning to give a drug involves four important steps. Match the process with each of the four steps.

32. _____ Know the major action of the drug.

33. _____ Learn what the drug is supposed to do for the patient.

34. _____ Learn whether the drug should be refrigerated.

35. _____ What does the patient need to know to take the drug correctly?

36. _____ What does the patient need to know about potential side effects?

37. _____ Learn whether the drug should be kept at room temperature.

38. _____ Learn the main drug interactions.

39. _____ Learn the usual dosage, route, and frequency.

1. Know the reason you are giving the patient the drug.
2. Learn specific information about the drug.
3. Plan for special storage or procedures, techniques, or equipment needs.
4. Develop a teaching plan for the patient.

List one component of safe drug administration for each of the nine rights of administration.

40. How do you ensure that you identify the right patient?

_____

41. How do you ensure that you are giving the right drug?

_____

42. How do you ensure that you are giving the drug at the right time?

_____

43. Who indicates the right dose of the drug you are giving?

_____

44. How do you know the right route to give the drug?

_____

45. Why does the right reason matter when giving the drug?

_____

46. How do you make sure you provide the right documentation?

_____

47. What must you do after the drug administration to ensure that the patient has the right response?

_____

48. How do you manage the patient's right to refuse a particular administration of a drug?

_____

3

PRACTICE QUIZ

1. Which one of the factors listed below has increased the demand for LPNs/VNs?
   a. There are an increased number of people who request LPNs/VNs.
   b. There are an increased number of people who are living with chronic illnesses.
   c. There are an increased number of people who need home healthcare.
   d. There are an increased number of people who are on fixed incomes.

2. LPN/VN practice has shifted over the past decade. Although currently most graduates practice in long-term and community-based settings, previously where did LPN/VNs most frequently practice?
   a. LPN/VNs practiced mostly in acute care settings (hospital-based care).
   b. LPN/VNs practiced mostly in healthcare clinics.
   c. LPN/VNs practiced mostly in healthcare provider's offices.
   d. LPN/VNs practiced mostly in schools.

3. What percentage of a work week does an LPN/VN usually spend giving drugs to patients and monitoring their reactions?
   a. 40% of the work week
   b. 25% of the work week
   c. 5% of the work week
   d. 50% of the work week

4. The nursing process guides your work when giving drugs. What are the five steps that are included in the process?
   a. History, Monitoring, Administering, Charting, and Assessment
   b. Assessment, Diagnosis, Planning, Implementation, and Evaluation
   c. Planning, Documenting, Screening, Diagnosing, and Administering
   d. Assessment, Administering, Documenting, Planning, and Monitoring

5. Why is it important to do a patient's history when he or she enters the healthcare setting?
   a. You must determine whether the patient is in the appropriate place.
   b. You will be able to assess the patient's ability to afford healthcare.
   c. You will provide the healthcare providers with information they need to identify physical signs of illness.
   d. You must diagnose the patient's illness before admitting the patient.

6. When doing a patient history, you will gather objective and subjective data. Why is this important information to gather on the patient?
   a. It can be used as a baseline for comparison of the patient's condition as care progresses.
   b. You can prove that you are completely knowledgeable of the patient's condition.
   c. You can tell whether the patient's information is accurate by comparing the objective to the subjective data.
   d. You are only responsible for monitoring subjective data.

7. Why is it important to ask what kinds of over-the-counter drugs a patient is taking?
   a. To ensure the patient continues taking them once he or she is admitted
   b. To identify potential interactions with any drugs the healthcare provider may prescribe
   c. To explain to the patient why taking over-the-counter drugs is not safe
   d. To determine if the patient is reacting to an over-the-counter drug

8. Although it is not your role to develop a medical or nursing diagnosis of the patient, what will you be responsible for?
   a. You will verify if the diagnosis is correct.
   b. You will not have any responsibilities once a diagnosis is made.
   c. You will decide how carefully the patient needs monitoring.
   d. You will decide when the drug must be given.

9. After giving the drug, you notice the patient's condition has improved. What is this effect named?
   a. Expected side effect
   b. Placebo effect
   c. Favorable effect
   d. Therapeutic effect

10. Which of the following tasks will you do as part of your continuing assessment of the patient to evaluate the effectiveness of the drug you are giving?
    a. Take the patient's blood pressure.
    b. Question the family about any improvements they have noticed.
    c. Review the chart to ensure the RN is documenting any changes.
    d. Determine if you think the drug prescribed was the appropriate choice.

11. If your patient refuses a drug, what is the best response?
    a. Inform the patient that taking the drug is mandatory.
    b. Contact the prescribing healthcare provider to discuss this with the patient.
    c. Find an online article for the patient to read.
    d. Explain the reason for the drug and answer any questions the patient has.

12. When documenting the administration of the drug, which of the following must you record in the patient's chart?
    a. The time the drug was supposed to be given
    b. The time the patient requested the drug be given
    c. The time the drug was given
    d. The time the drug was left with the patient

13. What is the preferred route of drug administration?
    a. Intravenous
    b. Intramuscular
    c. Oral
    d. Inhaler

14. Your 25-year-old female patient is given an antibiotic. What is one possible drug interaction that you should identify for this patient?
    a. You should ensure the patient is not using illegal drugs that would decrease the potency of the antibiotic.
    b. You should find out if the patient is using birth control pills and warn her that the antibiotic could interfere with the pill's effectiveness.
    c. You should find out if the patient drinks alcohol and warn her about possible interactions.
    d. You should find out if the patient will be adherent to taking the drug as ordered.

15. Before giving a drug, you must read the label three times. Which of the following is NOT one of the times you need to read the label?
    a. Read the label before taking the drug from the storage area.
    b. Read the label before preparing the prescribed dose of the drug.
    c. Read the label before opening the drug when giving it to the patient.
    d. Read the label before disposing of the packaging.

2 Legal, Regulatory, and Ethical Aspects of Drug Administration

MATCHING

Match the term associated with the situation described.

1. _____ Your patient refuses to take his drug so you decide to crush his pills and mix them in his oatmeal. However, you must inform him or his family of your method of getting him to take his pills.

2. _____ Before you crush his pills, however, you refer to the Institute of Safe Medicine website to ensure the pill can be used in this way.

3. _____ You suspect that one of your colleagues is actually not providing his patient all the drugs ordered for her pain. Instead the nurse is using a portion of the drugs for his own personal use.

4. _____ The nurse who is taking the pain drug is violating the American Nurse Association (ANA) Code of Ethics and is unable to fulfill his duties in a safe and effective manner.

5. _____ By utilizing these drugs for himself, this nurse has violated specific laws and may face fines or imprisonment.

6. _____ Before giving your patient a prescribed drug, it is important that you are familiar with possible reactions, the patient's current history, and whether the patient is responding appropriately.

A. Do not crush list
B. Impaired nurse
C. Covert drug administration
D. Nursing process
E. Controlled substance
F. Drug diversion

CONTROLLED SUBSTANCES

7. Some drugs are identified as controlled substances because there is a greater potential for their abuse than most prescription drugs. Controlled substances are categorized I through V based on their potential for abuse. From the list below, identify the schedule designation (I, II, III, IV, or V) of each drug.

_____ Tylenol #4

_____ Heroin

_____ Fiorinal

_____ Lomotil

_____ Ritalin

_____ Lysergic Acid Diethylamide

_____ Ativan

_____ Percodan

_____ Valium

_____ Promethazine

FILL IN THE BLANKS

8. As an LPN/LVN, you can dispense controlled substances only if permitted by your _____ board of nursing.

9. Scheduled drugs must be _____ at the end of every shift by the nurse whom the agency has given the responsibility for controlled substances.

10. Dosages of controlled substances are dispensed by the pharmacy with an accompanying _____ sheet on which the nurse must record the administration of the drug.

11. Drugs to be used for patients are kept either in a _____ cabinet or an automated dispensing system.

12. Access to these drugs is never given to _____ or any other unauthorized healthcare workers.

TRUE OF FALSE

13. Indicate with a T (true) or F (false) what information a legal prescription order must contain.

    _____ the patient's initials   _____ dose

    _____ prescriber's birthdate   _____ time prescription was ordered

    _____ name of drug   _____ duration

    _____ route of administration   _____ signature of pharmacist

MATCHING

Match the situation with the type of drug order that is applicable.

14. _____ A patient requires a daily dose of losartan for her blood pressure.

15. _____ A patient has an allergic reaction to a new drug that has just been given for the first time.

16. _____ A patient is given nitroglycerin just before undergoing a cardiac CT scan.

17. _____ A patient is given Tylenol #3 whenever she complains of intermittent pain.

A. Emergency or STAT drug order
B. As-needed drug order
C. Single drug order
D. Standing drug order

CONTROLLED SUBSTANCES

18. At the end of the shift, the controlled substance drug inventory does not account for all the dosages received for the shift. List at least three steps to try and account for the differences.

    _____

    _____

    _____

19. If you believe there has been an error in the administration of any drug, list at least three steps you should take to ensure the patient's safety.

    _____

    _____

    _____

PRACTICE QUIZ

1. As a nurse, you must learn about and follow three levels of rules in giving drugs. What entity is the first level that takes precedence over the remaining entities?
   a. International rules
   b. Agency (hospital or clinic) rules
   c. Federal rules
   d. State rules

2. Federal laws define three categories of drugs, including controlled substances and prescription drugs. What is the third category?
   a. Over-the-counter drugs
   b. Antibiotic drugs
   c. Steroid drugs
   d. Illegal drugs

3. A patient who has been taking controlled substances for pain decides she no longer needs them. After a few days, she begins shaking and becomes confused. What is this condition?
   a. Psychological dependence on the controlled substance
   b. Lack of pain control due to withholding drugs
   c. Method for gaining attention of healthcare provider
   d. Physical dependence resulting in drug withdrawal

4. Which of the following behaviors would lead you to suspect a coworker may be diverting controlled substances for her own personal use?
   a. She is unusually pleasant during her shift.
   b. Her work ethic is not up to the institution's standard.
   c. She frequently reports dropping or spilling controlled substances.
   d. She is snacking more frequently during her shift.

5. Your patients has just been prescribed a new drug that you are instructed to give. This patient has had a number of bad reactions to drugs so as part of your due diligence, what will you do to reduce the risk of an adverse reaction to the new drug?
   a. Ensure that the drug will not react poorly with any other drugs she is already taking.
   b. Give the drug as prescribed, as the physician would be aware of possible interactions.
   c. Avoid providing the drug until your nursing supervisor ensures it is safe.
   d. Crush the drug and mix it with her coffee so she will not object to additional drugs.

6. When entering the room of a patient under your care at an assisted living facility, you discover he is swallowing several doses of Tylenol. What should be your response?
   a. Report the incident immediately to his physician in case of adverse reactions.
   b. Remove the Tylenol and explain to the patient that he cannot take any drugs including over-the-counter drugs, without his healthcare provider's written permission.
   c. Distract the patient, then remove the bottle of Tylenol and dispose of it based on your institution's policy for disposal of drugs.
   d. Contact the patient's family and inform them that he will not be permitted to remain on the premises if he continues to disobey the institution's policy on over-the-counter drugs.

7. You cannot give a drug unless there is a prescription ordered by a healthcare provider who has prescription authority. Who of the following individuals would most likely NOT have authority to sign a prescription?
   a. Nurse practitioner
   b. Physician's assistant
   c. Psychologist
   d. Dentist

8. After moving halfway across the country to another state, you are ready to start work again but have a few questions about what the state allows you as an LPN/LVN to do regarding the administration of drugs. You want to find out the Nurse Practice Act for your new home. Where would you find this information?
   a. National Council of State Boards of Nursing (NCSBN) website
   b. The official state website regarding licensing and renewal of licenses for all healthcare providers
   c. The state capitol library that houses all documents relating to healthcare practice
   d. A brochure from the ANA

9. Why does an electronic health record that has the capability of scanning a patient's wristband provide more accuracy when identifying a patient?
   a. You will avoid having to complete an inventory sheet
   b. The responsibility is shifted to the nurse leader for your shift
   c. You will avoid having to decipher illegible handwriting
   d. There is no possibility of losing the patient's record

10. Drug errors most commonly occur at which of the following points in drug administration?
    a. During drug preparation
    b. When bringing the drug to the patient
    c. When giving the drug to the patient
    d. All of the above
    e. A and C only

11. Almost everyone makes an error at some point in his or her career. Which of the following situations could make a nurse more reluctant to report the error?
    a. The nurse is afraid people will think he or she is diverting drugs for personal use.
    b. The nurses license is automatically suspended for an indefinite period.
    c. The agency is unusually harsh and judgmental about drug errors among nurses.
    d. Nurses fear being sued by the patient or his family.

12. What does the **black box warning** on the inset of the drug packaging indicate?
    a. The drug is highly addictive, and most patients will be at a higher risk for dependency.
    b. The drug has a higher-than-normal risk for causing serious and even life-threatening problems.
    c. The drug is experimental, and unusual reactions may occur in many patients
    d. The drug has been packaged in another country and may be contaminated.

13. Which of the following practices can cause the most potential harm when caring for a patient with a communicable disease?
    a. Recapping a needle that you just used to inject the patient
    b. Touching any part of the patient without first donning gloves
    c. Removing soiled linens and not disposing of them properly
    d. Not wearing a mask at all times when you are in contact with the patient

14. In the acronym PINCH, P is for potassium, I is for insulin, N is for narcotics (opioids), C is for cancer chemotherapy drugs, and H is for heparin or any drug type that interferes with blood clotting. This acronym is helpful for identifying which category of drugs?
    a. Prescription drugs
    b. High-alert drugs
    c. Refrigerated drugs
    d. Specialized drugs

15. Why might you not be able to crush a particular drug and give it to one of your patients who has difficulty swallowing the drug?
    a. Mixing the drug with food can generate toxins.
    b. The patient's family has expressly indicated that this method is unacceptable as it will seem as if the patient's dignity is in question.
    c. Crushing the drug will speed up the delivery to the patient's system, which may create adverse reactions.
    d. Your institution has a policy forbidding this type of drug administration.

KEY WORDS IN PHARMACOLOGY

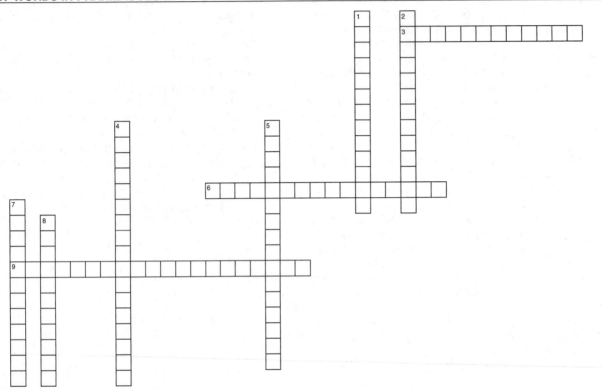

ACROSS

3. Drug that may replace another drug at a receptor site, decreasing the effect of the first drug
6. What the drug does to the body
9. The use of drugs in the treatment of disease

DOWN

1. Products that are chemically the same
2. Reponses to a drug that are strange, unique, peculiar, or unpredicted
4. Process that happens mainly in the liver where there are enzymes that break down the chemicals that make up the drug into its usable and unusable parts
5. What the body does to the drug
7. Patients may see several specialists, each of whom may prescribe different drugs
8. These drugs have the potential to cause birth defects

MATCHING

Match the descriptions with the drug name. You may use an answer more than once.

_____ 10. Drug name followed by the symbol ®, which indicates that the name is registered to a specific drug maker

_____ 11. Most common name used for a drug

_____ 12. Name used for a drug that is the same throughout the world

_____ 13. Names that include all the different substances used to make the drug

_____ 14. The proprietary name of a drug

A. Generic name
B. Trade/Brand name
C. Chemical name

FILL IN THE BLANK

15. Indicate whether the drug action described below identifies it as an agonist, partial agonist, or antagonist.
    A. In the case of an opiate overdose, Naloxone is given to a patient to reverse the effects of the opiate, which is bound to the opioid receptor sites. _____

    B. A patient is in severe pain and is given morphine, which then activates the opioid receptors and produces pain relief. _____

    C. Buspirone is given to a patient who is already taking Prozac to help boost the effects of the antidepressant. _____

16. The _____ process identifies how the drug enters the body and reaches the area it needs to affect.

17. Absorption of a drug is enabled through the processes of diffusion, _____, and osmosis.

18. Before a drug can enter the body's tissues, it must be dissolved in body fluid. How effectively a drug can dissolve is called _____.

19. Upon entering the body, the drug must reach the area needing treatment. The method of movement can occur by way of the blood or lymph system and is known as _____ of the drug.

20. Biotransformation is the process by which the body transforms the drug into usable or inactive components and happens primarily in the _____.

21. List five methods that can be used to give drugs to a patient.

_____

_____

_____

_____

_____

MULTIPLE SELECTION

22. Excretion is the process of removing the inactive chemicals, by-products, and waste from the body. From the list below, check each of the methods by which chemicals are excreted.
    ☐ Fecal matter
    ☐ Saliva
    ☐ Hair follicles
    ☐ Urine
    ☐ Bathing

11

☐ Sweating
☐ Crying
☐ Nail growth
☐ Weight loss

MATCHING

23. Indicate whether the following responses by a patient who has been given one or more drugs are more likely to be (A) side effects or (B) adverse reactions.

_____ Sleepiness

_____ Anaphylactic shock

_____ Seizures

_____ Nausea

_____ Bleeding

_____ Diarrhea

_____ Constipation

_____ Kidney damage

SHORT ANSWER

24. Describe one drug therapy difference between African American persons and white persons.

25. Explain why individuals may require different dosages of the same drug.

26. Why do individuals with liver or kidney problems usually need smaller, less frequent dosages?

27. How does body size affect the dosages prescribed for individuals?

MATCHING

It is important to identify the characteristics associated with the life stage of the patient. Match the characteristic with the life stage.

_____ 28. Drug side effects more severe

_____ 29. Highest metabolism of all age groups

_____ 30. Oral drugs poorly absorbed

_____ 31. Growth spurts increase metabolism

_____ 32. Higher percentage of total body water

_____ 33. Dehydrates more easily

_____ 34. Poor intramuscular absorption

_____ 35. Hypotension

A. Older adults
B. Newborns/Infants
C. Adolescents
D. Children

PRACTICE QUIZ

1. In order to avoid confusion over the various names given to drugs, many hospitals are now using which of the following drug names, which is the most common name and is recognized all over the world?
   a. Trade name
   b. Generic name
   c. Chemical name
   d. Proprietary name

2. *Ethyl 1-methyl-4-phenyl isonipecotate hydrochloride* is an example of which of the following drug names?
   a. Trade name
   b. Generic name
   c. Chemical name
   d. Proprietary name

3. For a drug to work inside the body, it needs to attach to which of the following areas in order to activate the chemical reaction between the drug and the body?
   a. Nerve cells
   b. Receptor sites
   c. Liver
   d. Mitochondria

4. Your patient is experiencing pain, and it is not yet time for her next dose of pain reliever. What can you do to help her decrease the pain without the use of drugs?
   a. Massage her neck for several minutes to help her relax.
   b. Distract her with television or read to her.
   c. Get her to try simple yoga exercises in bed to help her stretch.
   d. Encourage her to do deep breathing to release the body's own endorphins.

5. Mr. B, a 78-year-old patient, is given a capsule to swallow, and you encourage him to drink a full cup of water with the pill. Why is this important?
   a. You suspect he is dehydrated, and the water will help the drug dissolve and begin working in the body more quickly.
   b. You are afraid that without enough water, Mr. B will choke on the capsule.
   c. The capsule has a strong taste that will be unpleasant to Mr. B and may make him reluctant to take his next dose.
   d. It is standard hospital policy that all patients consume a cup of water with oral drugs.

6. Mrs. X takes a Valium every night before sleeping. However, she has a very difficult time waking in the morning. When you report this to her healthcare provider, why does she replace the Valium with Ativan?
   a. The healthcare provider suspects an adverse reaction to Valium.
   b. Valium should not be used for more than 2 to 3 days.
   c. Valium stays longer in the body because it builds up in fat cells.
   d. The healthcare provider suspects the patient may be becoming addicted to Valium.

7. A patient in your care is being treated for high blood pressure. You note, however, that the drug is not as effective as expected, so you discuss it with your patient. Discovery of which of the following would indicate a need for increased dosage?
   a. The patient must take the drug twice a day and usually forgets the second dose.
   b. The patient is dehydrated, and the drug is not being distributed effectively.
   c. The patient has untreated sleep apnea and therefore needs additional drugs.
   d. The patient did not report having liver disease, and therefore the drug is not effectively delivered throughout the body.

Chapter **3 Principles of Pharmacology**

8. Mr. Y reports having only one kidney due to a bad infection during childhood. Why is this important to know when monitoring his reaction to a new drug?
   a. Mr. Y may be prone to infections, and therefore it is important to identify any symptoms that indicate an infection may be developing.
   b. Mr. Y's decreased kidney function may indicate that the drug is not being excreted effectively, and he may experience an overdose of the drug.
   c. The kidney loss may impact the ability of the body to dissolve the drug in a timely manner.
   d. Kidney damage is listed as a possible adverse reaction of the drug, so it is vital to ensure his kidney is functioning effectively.

9. A patient appears to be overdosed but insists she only took the amount of long-acting drug as prescribed and followed all other instructions. Upon further questioning, you discover which of the following as the likely reason for her reaction?
   a. She experiences difficulty swallowing and therefore crushed the tablet and ate it with her morning bowl of oatmeal.
   b. She is overweight, and the drug has built up in her fat cells.
   c. She usually takes the drug with an alcoholic beverage, which is contraindicated on the package.
   d. She has a very slow metabolism, and the drug stayed too long in her system.

10. Which of the following is a *paradoxical response* to a drug that should be monitored?
    a. The patient takes Benedryl and becomes drowsy.
    b. The patient takes an aspirin, and her nose begins to bleed.
    c. The patient takes a steroid, and his level of energy increases.
    d. The patient is on chemotherapy for breast cancer and feels nauseous.

11. Of all the factors listed below that can impact the safety and effectiveness of a drug, which one is most commonly attributed to life-threatening adverse reactions?
    a. Drug–food interactions
    b. Drug–alcohol interactions
    c. Drug–tobacco interactions
    d. Drugs that interact adversely with other drugs, including over-the-counter drugs

12. Why is it important to note whether your patient is dehydrated or overhydrated when adjusting the dosage of a new prescription?
    a. Hydration impacts the blood flow, which determines how well the drug is distributed throughout the body.
    b. Proper hydration reduces the chance for adverse reactions to a drug.
    c. Some drugs react adversely to water.
    d. Hydration can impact metabolism, which controls the distribution of the drug to the liver.

13. What is one reason that it is important for you to know as much as possible about a drug before giving it to your patient?
    a. If you are not familiar with all the names, you may give the incorrect drug.
    b. You will need to report at the end of your shift all the drugs you have given.
    c. You will need to know the most common side effects and observe for adverse reactions in each of your patients, particularly when giving a drug for the first time.
    d. You are legally required to identify all drugs by generic and chemical names before giving them to a patient.

14. One of your patients has just been given a new prescription. However, she explains to you that she is currently nursing her newborn. What is one way to help reduce adversely impacting her baby with the drug?
    a. You can advise her to avoid taking the drug and try natural methods to reduce her symptoms.
    b. You assure her that the drug cannot be passed to the baby while she is nursing.
    c. You recommend she take the drug immediately after nursing so that it has a chance to be excreted before nursing time again.
    d. You suggest weaning the infant and moving to formula.

15. You have been instructed to give an intramuscular injection to a 5-year-old child. To ensure rapid absorption, which of the following muscles is the best place to give the injection?
    a. Gluteal
    b. Deltoid
    c. Vastus lateralis
    d. Rectus abdominis

4 Drug Calculation: Preparing and Giving Drugs

CALCULATION

1. Your patient has an order for 500 mg of amoxicillin. The pharmacy sends you 250-mg capsules. Using the dimensional analysis method, what is the correct number of capsules to give your patient?

2. The healthcare provider has ordered 0.5 g of amoxicillin oral suspension for your patient. The pharmacy sends you the drug with instructions stating that 1 teaspoon is equal to 250 mg. Using the fraction method, calculate how many teaspoons to give to your patient.

3. You are to give 180 mg of Lasix to your patient. You have received 40-mg tablets. Using the ratio and proportion method, how many tablets do you give your patient?

4. Your patient needs 80 mg of lisinopril. The pharmacy has provided you with 20-mg tablets. Using all three methods (dimensional analysis, fraction, and ratio and proportion), how many tablets do you give to your patient?

5. What is the correct equipment to use in giving 80 units of insulin detemir?

6. Amoxicillin, 500 mg, is a typical adult dosage. Using Clark's rule, what is the correct dosage for a 10-year-old boy who weighs 70 pounds?

MATCHING

Match the definition or calculation with the appropriate intravenous administration term. You may use each term more than once.

7. _____ How fast the IV infuses

8. _____ (Total drops to be infused/Flow rate) x 60 drops/hour

9. _____ Number of drops used to make a mL of IV fluid

10. _____ Drop factor X milliliters/minute = Flow rate (drops/minute)

11. _____ Differs by manufacturer

12. _____ Depends on the total number of drops, amount of fluid, and the number of minutes the IV is to flow

A. Infusion time
B. Drop factor
C. Flow rate

IDENTIFICATION: MACRODRIP AND MICRODRIP

For each drop factor listed below, indicate whether the tubing that should be used is macrodrip (a) or microdrip (b).

13. _____ 10 drops/mL

14. _____ 15 drops/mL

15. _____ 20 drops/mL

16. _____ 60 drops/mL

17. _____ Used most often for children and elderly patients

18. _____ Used most often when faster infusion rates are needed

MATCHING

Match the descriptions below with the appropriate term that identifies drug types or administration routes. Use each term only once.

19. _____ Drugs given directly into the GI tract

20. _____ Drugs that must be shaken before administration

21. _____ Drugs applied to the skin or mucous membranes (e.g., topicals, patches, or ear drops)

22. _____ Method used to inject between the skin and the muscle layer

23. _____ Has two compartments that contain a sterile solution and a drug powder separated by a rubber stopper

24. _____ Method that seals the injection site and prevents leakage of the drug

25. _____ Method used to inject between the upper two layers of skin

26. _____ Drug administration that bypasses the mouth by use of a tube that goes through nose and esophagus into the stomach

27. _____ Method used when the drug ordered may be destroyed by gastric enzymes

28. _____ Method used to deposit deep into the muscle mass

A. Nasogastric tube
B. Parenteral route
C. Enteral drugs
E. Liquid-form oral drugs
F. Intramuscular route
G. Mix-O-Vial
H. Intradermal route
I. Subcutaneous route
J. Z-track technique
K. Percutaneous route

SAFETY CONSIDERATIONS

Answer the following questions about drug administration safety.

29. Before giving tablets or capsules, make sure the patient is able to do what?

30. To ensure a drug is evenly distributed throughout a liquid before giving, what must be done first?

31. Why is insulin considered a high-alert drug?

32. When a patient is unable to swallow a tablet or capsule, why must you check with the pharmacist before crushing tablets or breaking capsules?

33. What are some steps you can take to assist a patient who has difficulty swallowing the drug?

34. Why should you give drugs separately through a nasogastric (NG) or percutaneous endoscopic gastrostomy (PEG) tube?

35. When giving a drug subcutaneously, why should you avoid aspiration?

36. The preferred IM injection sites are deltoid, vastus lateralis, and ventrogluteal muscles. Why is the dorsogluteal muscle **NOT** recommended?

37. When a patient is receiving intravenous drugs, what are some observations you should make to ensure the patient's safety?

38. When giving topical or transdermal drugs, why should you avoid touching the drugs with your bare hands or fingers?

PRACTICE QUIZ

1. Although many drugs are currently prepackaged at the correct dosage, what is at least one reason to know how to accurately calculate correct drug dosage?
   a. You need to ensure the pharmacy did not send you the incorrect dosage.
   b. The drug dosage ordered is not available in the pharmacy.
   c. Patients may ask you to ensure the dosage is correct.
   d. Some institutions require that you show calculations have been made before giving the drug.

2. How does The Joint Commission, a nonprofit agency that credentials and certifies healthcare organizations, currently recommend that all drug dosages for children be calculated?
   a. Weight-based
   b. Age-based
   c. Height-based
   d. Activity-based

3. What is a major disadvantage of giving IV drugs that enter the bloodstream directly?
   a. Patients may experience discomfort being attached to an IV.
   b. IV administration requires more time in monitoring the patient.
   c. IV administration of a drug is often more complex, and there is more possibility of an error in dosages.
   d. The potential for adverse events that range from allergic reactions to death is higher.

4. Which of the following is a basic guide for giving any type of drug to your patient?
   a. Always wash your hands before giving a drug to avoid contamination.
   b. You should always recap syringes after giving a patient an injection.
   c. Unwrap and remove drugs from containers before you are with the patient.
   d. If the patient is sleeping or otherwise engaged, leave the drug with the patient to take at his or her convenience.

17

5. What is a disadvantage of giving oral drugs?
   a. Tablets resist the acidic pH of the stomach.
   b. Oral drugs are inconvenient.
   c. Oral drugs are more expensive than other types of drugs.
   d. Some oral drugs become ineffective when coming in contact with the acid and enzymes in the intestines.

6. How are drugs given through a nasogastric tube (NG)?
   a. Tube going directly through the throat into the stomach
   b. Tube going through the nose and esophagus into the stomach
   c. Tube going directly through the abdomen wall into the stomach
   d. Tube going through the chest wall into the stomach

7. What is the best way to ensure the NG tube is most likely in the stomach?
   a. Auscultation over the stomach and listening for a "whooshing" sound
   b. Patient able to take deep breaths
   c. Testing the pH of the stomach contents to ensure it is 0-5
   d. Aspirating some stomach content and ensuring you identify undigested food

8. What is one common reason for giving drugs intravenously?
   a. Patient has a severe infection.
   b. Patient has allergic reaction to oral drugs.
   c. Patient is unconscious and not likely to object to IV placement.
   d. Patient needs drug to act more slowly.

9. Which of the following is true about syringes?
   a. Syringes are available in only one size.
   b. Calibrations are printed numbers on the barrel of the syringe and indicate the amount of drug.
   c. The plunger is the portion of the syringe that holds the needle.
   d. The tip of the syringe is removed before giving an injection.

10. When using a vial that contains parenteral drugs, what is one step you should use when filling a syringe with the solution?
    a. Inject air equal to solution amount into the vial.
    b. Do not clean the rubber diaphragm across the top of the glass container before inserting the needle.
    c. Do not remove the metal lid from the glass container.
    d. Insert the needle into the vial bevel down.

11. Which of the following types of containers requires a filter needle to draw up the drug?
    a. Mix-O-Vial
    b. Multiple dose vial
    c. Ampule
    d. Cartridge

12. Why are intradermal injections usually made in the inner forearm, scapular area, or the upper chest?
    a. These areas are less sensitive.
    b. The blood supply to these areas is less.
    c. There is quicker absorption from the intradermal layer.
    d. The skin area has more hair and hides the injection site.

13. Where are subcutaneous injections given?
    a. Between the two upper layers of the skin
    b. Between the muscle layer and the fat layer
    c. Between the dermis of the skin and the muscle layer
    d. Between the lower layers of the skin

14. What is one of the primary reasons for giving drugs through the intramuscular route?
    a. Muscles are larger and therefore cause less pain to the patient.
    b. You have more locations to rotate injections.
    c. Allows for slower drug absorption.
    d. Allows for more rapid drug absorption.

15. If aspiration is required for an intramuscular injection, what action do you take if blood is drawn into the syringe?
    a. Try again until you no longer withdraw blood, then give the dose.
    b. Discard the drug and syringe and prepare a new dose.
    c. Withdraw the needle and massage the area of injection.
    d. Wait several hours and try again.

16. Which of the following muscles is **NOT** a recommended site for intramuscular injections?
    a. Dorsogluteal
    b. Deltoid
    c. Vastus lateralis
    d. Ventrogluteal

5 Anti-infective Drugs: Antibacterial, Antitubercular, and Antifungal Agents

IDENTIFYING TYPES OF DRUGS

Match the drug name with the category of drug(s). You may use categories more than once.

Drug Names

1. _____ azithromycin
2. _____ nystatin
3. _____ pyrazinamide
4. _____ fluconazole
5. _____ amoxicillin
6. _____ griseofulvin
7. _____ doxycycline
8. _____ metronidazole
9. _____ ethambutol
10. _____ praziquantel
11. _____ rifampin
12. _____ clindamycin
13. _____ ciprofloxacin
14. _____ streptomycin
15. _____ isoniazid
16. _____ cefuroxime
17. _____ pyrazinamide
18. _____ sulfamethoxazole/trimethoprim
19. _____ cefazolin
20. _____ linezolid
21. _____ imipenem
22. _____ erythromycin
23. _____ chloroquine

Drug Categories

A. Penicillins
B. Cephalosporins
C. Carbapenems
D. Tetracyclines
E. Macrolides
F. Aminoglycosides
G. Miscellaneous protein synthesis inhibitors
H. Sulfonamides
I. Fluoroquinolones
J. First-line drug therapies for tuberculosis
K. Common antifungal drugs
L. Common antiparasitic drugs

SHORT ANSWER

24. List at least three disease-producing pathogens that can cause an infection.

19

25. Name two reasons why it is important for you to learn as much as possible about anti-infective drugs.

26. Organisms are located throughout most of our bodies and are referred to as normal flora. What can happen when the normal flora is disrupted by antibiotic treatment?

27. When antibiotics are overused, or used incorrectly, what is the possible outcome?

28. The Center for Disease Control (CDC) identifies 18 drug-resistant threats in the United States. Which three are considered urgent?

29. To improve the effectiveness of existing drugs, newer, more focused drugs are continually being developed. How are these newer drugs identified by healthcare professionals?

DRUG ACTIONS

Match the drug action with the category of drug(s). You may use categories more than once and some drug actions will include multiple categories.

Drug Action

30. _____ Treats fungal or mycotic infections

31. _____ Interferes with the creation and repair of bacterial cell walls

32. _____ Prevents bacteria from making the final form of folic acid needed to metabolize

33. _____ Affects the function of DNA and/or RNA to kill protozoan parasites

34. _____ Controls *M. tuberculosis* bacteria and prevents its spread to various organ systems

35. _____ Interferes with processes used by the bacterium to make proteins needed for growth

36. _____ Inhibits cell wall synthesis

37. _____ Destroys bacteria by inhibiting enzymes needed for DNA synthesis and reproduction

Drug Categories

A. Penicillins
B. Cephalosporins
C. Carbapenems
D. Tetracyclines
E. Macrolides
F. Aminoglycosides
G. Sulfonamides
H. Fluoroquinolones
I. First-line drug therapies for tuberculosis
J. Common antifungal drugs
K. Common antiparasitic drugs

20

MULTIPLE CHOICE

For each of the drug types listed below, check all the statements that are applicable.

Penicillin

38. _____ Used for *prophylactic* treatment against bacterial endocarditis in patients with rheumatic or heart disease before dental procedures or surgery.

39. _____ The most common side effect is sinus congestion.

40. _____ Allergic reactions occur in 2–5% of the population, producing rash, *erythema* (redness or inflammation), *urticaria* (hives), *angioedema* (swelling of the skin and mucous membranes), *laryngeal edema* (swelling of the larynx), and *anaphylaxis* (shock).

Cephalosporins

41. _____ Used for uncomplicated skin and soft tissue infections; infections of the lower respiratory tract, central nervous system (CNS), genitourinary system, joints, and bones; and for serious infections, such as bacteremia and septicemia.

42. _____ Nausea, vomiting, and diarrhea are frequent but usually mild.

43. _____ The most common adverse effect is tinnitus.

Vancomycin and Carbapenems

44. _____ Never used for infections caused by multidrug-resistant (MDR) bacteria in hospitalized patients.

45. _____ Side effects and adverse effects are severe, so use of these drugs is generally limited to young adults who are not immune-compromised.

46. _____ An unusual response is a deep red rash on the upper body known as "red man syndrome" that is produced by a histamine-released reaction.

Tetracyclines

47. _____ First-choice drugs in incidents of MRSA.

48. _____ Side effects include mild episodes of nausea, vomiting, and diarrhea.

49. _____ May cause permanent damage (skeletal retardation) to a developing fetus.

Macrolides

50. _____ Alternatives to penicillin for patients with a penicillin allergy and for infections caused by organisms that are resistant to penicillin.

51. _____ Most common side effects include mild abdominal pain, nausea, flatulence.

52. _____ Can impair the liver and cause jaundice.

Aminoglycosides

53. _____ Treats serious aerobic gram-positive infections, including those caused by *Escherichia coli, Serratia, Proteus, Klebsiella*, and *Pseudomonas*.

54. _____ Intravenous administration can cause skin rashes.

55. _____ May damage the kidney *(nephrotoxicity)* and can produce permanent damage to the inner ear *(ototoxicity)* or hearing impairment.

Sulfonamides

56. _____ Used for treating acute and chronic urinary tract infections, particularly cystitis, pyelitis, and pyelonephritis.

57. _____ Side effects include *vertigo* (feeling of dizziness or spinning), *tinnitus* (ringing in the ears), hearing loss, and *stomatitis* (inflammation of the mouth).

58. _____ Can suppress bone marrow function, increasing the risk for anemia, bleeding, and reduced immunity.

Fluoroquinolones

59. _____ Effective against gram-negative pathogens.

60. _____ Common side effects are secondary infections.

61. _____ *Arthropathy* (joint pain and disease) can occur, especially in children.

Antitubercular Drugs

62. _____ Used to control the active disease and prevent its spread to various organ systems in the infected patient or to other people.

63. _____ Side effects include nausea, vomiting, diarrhea, headache, and sleeplessness.

64. _____ Causes cardiovascular incidents.

Antifungal Drugs

65. _____ Used orally, intravenously, topically, and vaginally to treat a variety of viral infections.

66. _____ Nausea, vomiting, and diarrhea are the most common expected side effects.

67. _____ Adverse reactions are associated with more severe problems such as toxicity to the neurlogic, cardiac, hematologic, liver, and renal systems.

Antiparasitic Drugs

68. _____ Inhibits DNA and RNA enzymes and decreases the pH inside the parasite so it is able to use the hemoglobin in the human red blood cells.

69. _____ May cause nosebleed and depression.

70. _____ Optic neuritis can occur with symptoms of eye pain or vision changes, and permanent vision loss can occur.

Anthelmintics

71. _____ Used in destroying worms that enter the body, usually through contaminated water or food.

72. _____ Nausea, vomiting, headache, abdominal pain, and drowsiness are common side effects.

73. _____ Praziquantel can worsen symptoms of arthritis.

FILL IN THE BLANKS

For the following general teaching information for antimicrobial drugs, fill in the blank(s) with the appropriate word(s).

74. Ordinary _____ is an expected side effect. However, excessive watery and bloody _____ with severe abdominal pain and fever is a complication and needs to be reported to the prescriber immediately.

75. If the patient develops a _____ in the throat, difficulty breathing, or swelling of the lips, tongue, or throat, call 911 immediately.

76. Instruct patients to take antimicrobial drugs exactly as _____ to prevent infection recurrence and drug resistance.

77. Instruct patients to stop taking the drug and notify the healthcare provider if a rash or hives develop while taking an antimicrobial drug. A drug _____ can develop at any time after the patient begins treatment.

78. Remind patients to report any new _____ that occur while taking antimicrobial therapy to the healthcare provider because they may represent an adverse reaction.

79. Tell patients that even though it may be inconvenient to take a drug in the middle of the night, it is important to space the drugs out _____ during the 24 hours for best results.

80. Instruct patients not to save antimicrobial drugs because many out-of-date drugs _____ and become less effective.

PRACTICE QUIZ

1. Which of the following descriptions **best** identifies infections?
   a. An overproduction of the body's normal flora that upsets the pH balance of the tissue
   b. Invasion of tissue by disease-producing pathogens that multiply and produce toxins
   c. Invasion of the body of parasitical bacteria that disrupts the ability of the body to produce antibodies
   d. Disruption of the body's existing microbiome, which invades the tissue and organs

2. How do antibiotics impact the normal flora of the body?
   a. Antibiotic use strengthens the normal flora balance in the body.
   b. Normal flora of the body can impact the ability of antibiotics to destroy or weaken bacterial infections.
   c. Normal flora protects the body from damage by antibiotics.
   d. Antibiotics can kill off the normal flora, causing yeast or fungal infections.

3. Why are gram-negative bacteria more difficult to treat than gram-positive bacteria?
   a. The cell wall is more complex with an outer capsule and two cell wall membranes.
   b. Gram-positive bacteria have a thin cell wall and no outer capsule.
   c. Gram-negative bacteria have developed resistance to most first-generation antibiotics.
   d. Gram-positive bacteria have poorly formed cellular structures.

4. Which of the following organisms is a common human parasite?
   a. Mycosis
   b. Nectotrophs
   c. Helminthes
   d. Streptococcus viridans

5. What is a superbug or a multidrug-resistant (MDR) organism?
   a. An organism resistant to three or more different types of antibiotic drugs
   b. An organism that is resistant to all antibiotic drugs and is usually treated through chemotherapy or surgery
   c. An organism that is resistant to penicillin
   d. Drug-resistant bacteria spread by birds and animals

6. If a female is taking oral contraceptives, what should you advise her to do if an antibiotic drug is prescribed?
   a. Review optional types of antibiotics with her prescriber that won't interfere with her contraceptive.
   b. Use another form of birth control during treatment to avoid contraception.
   c. Advise her to avoid sexual relations during drug therapy to prevent infecting her partner.
   d. Ensure her that antibiotics do not affect other drugs she may currently be taking, including oral contraceptives.

7. When taking strong antibiotics, patients could develop pseudomembranous colitis. What organism is responsible for this condition?
   a. *E. coli*
   b. *Helicobacter pylori*
   c. *Mycoplasma pneumoniae*
   d. Clo*stridium difficile*

8. Why should you always be aware of the start and stop dates of antimicrobial drugs such as aminoglycoside antibiotics?
   a. Excessive exposure can create adverse effects that permanently damage the patient's health.
   b. Excessive exposure can reduce effectiveness and increase chances the infection will return.
   c. Excessive exposure to antimicrobial drugs can create sterility in both men and women.
   d. Excessive exposure can increase the chances that the patient will develop an allergic reaction.

9. A major nursing responsibility with antimicrobial therapy is evaluating the effectiveness of the drug prescribed for the infection. Which action is necessary for evaluation of the patient's response to the antimicrobial therapy?
   a. Determine whether the patient is actually infected by looking for the typical symptoms of most bacterial infections.
   b. Observe whether symptoms improve 5 to 7 days after beginning drug therapy.
   c. Ensure the patient takes all the drug as prescribed, unless symptoms improve within 72 hours.
   d. Review laboratory work to ensure there are no adverse effects to the liver or kidneys.

10. What is the general cause of superinfections?
    a. Multiple infections requiring an array of drug therapies
    b. Tuberculosis that requires antimicrobial treatment for up to 6 months
    c. Antifungals given together with corticosteroid therapy, which reduces the immunity response
    d. Infections that are resistant to the majority of antibiotics currently on the market

23

6 Antivirals and Antiretrovirals

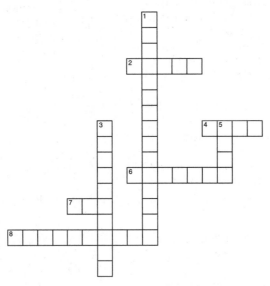

ACROSS

2. A small infection agent that can reproduce only inside other living cells, including human cells
4. A combination of antiretroviral drugs that must be taken every day to combat the progression of HIV disease from becoming AIDs
6. New viral particles reproduced in cells infected retroviruses that can leave the cell and infect more human body cells
7. Human Immunodeficiency Virus
8. Drugs capable of interfering with the ability of the virus to carry out its reproductive functions

DOWN

1. Drugs that are a subset of antiviral drugs and specifically suppress the reproduction of retroviruses
3. Viral organisms that carry special enzymes (reverse transcriptase, integrase, and protease) with them and use RNA (ribonuceleic acid) instead of DNA as their genes to reproduce
5. Acquired Immune Deficiency Syndrome

VIRUS OR RETROVIRUS

Indicate whether each of the statements below describes a Virus (V) or a Retrovirus (R).

9. _____ Infectious agent that reproduces only inside other living cells

10. _____ Causes damage and eventual death of an infected cell

11. _____ Transmits its own information into a cell's DNA

12. _____ Surrounded by a protein or fatty coating known as a capsid

13. _____ Uses the host cell's metabolic systems to make new viral particles

IDENTIFYING ANTIVIRAL DRUGS

Match the drug(s) used to treat each of the following viruses. (Some viruses may have more than one type of drug associated with treatment.)

Viruses

14. _____ Herpes

15. _____ Influenza

16. _____ Cytomegalovirus (CMV)

17. _____ Respiratory Syncytial Virus (RSV)

18. _____ Hepatitis B virus (HBV)

19. _____ Hepatitis C virus (HCV)

Drugs

A. Semeprevir
B. Adefovir
C. Famciclovir
D. Foscarnet
E. Ribavirin
F. Ledipasvir
G. Amantadine
H. Entecavir
I. Penciclovir

ANTIVIRAL SIDE EFFECTS & ADVERSE REACTIONS

Place an X next to each of the following items that identify a common (**NOT** adverse) side effect that you must look for when a patient is being treated with an antiviral drug.

20. _____ Vomiting

21. _____ Kidney damage

22. _____ Depression

23. _____ Diarrhea

24. _____ Headache

25. _____ Reddened skin (when using topicals)

List at least two adverse effects from common antiviral drugs that you need to monitor if your patient is being treated for one of the following viruses.

26. Flu _____

27. Herpes _____

28. CMV _____

29. RSV _____

30. HPB _____

31. HVC_____

TEACHING PATIENTS AND FAMILIES ABOUT ANTIVIRALS

Fill in the blank for each of the topics below that describe the type of information patients and their families need to be aware of when taking antiviral drugs.

32. If using _____ cream, warn them the skin may become red and excessive use can cause systemic side effects.

32. Be aware of true _____ allergies.

33. Expected side effects to _____ include vomiting, nausea, diarrhea, or headache.

34. When using topical drugs for treatment of HSV-1 (cold sores) or HSV-2 (genital herpes), use gloves and wash your

_____ thoroughly so the infection does not spread.

35. There is no cure for _____. Antivirals can only treat _____ prophylactically or symptomatically.

36. Check yourself (or your family member) _____ for worsening symptoms that may indicate pneumonia or bacterial infection.

37. Antivirals can also be used for prevention or prophylaxis of the _____ in unvaccinated persons who have been exposed to the disease.

38. Follow the specific _____ instructions for the drug listed on the package.

ANTIRETROVIRAL DRUGS MATCHING

Match the drug names with one of the six categories of antiretroviral therapy drugs. You may use the categories more than once.

Drugs

39. _____ Fosamprenavir

40. _____ Enfuvirtide

41. _____ Delavirdine

42. _____ Dolutegravir

43. _____ Abacavir

44. _____ Maraviroc

45. _____ Atazanavir

46. _____ Dolutegravir

47. _____ Efavirenz

Categories

A. Nucleoside reverse transcriptase inhibitors
B. Nonnucleoside reverse transcriptase inhibitors
C. Protease inhibitors
D. Integrase inhibitors
E. Fusion inhibitors
F. Entry inhibitors

Match each drug category with one or more cautions that patients and their families need to know about when taking drugs from that category. (Each caution may have more than one drug category associated with the action and categories can be used more than once.)

Cautions

48. _____ Do not chew or crush as this causes the drug to be absorbed too rapidly.

49. _____ Do not take if pregnant to avoid birth defects.

50. _____ Avoid St. John's Wort.

51. _____ Avoid fatty and fried foods.

52. _____ Take at least 1 hour before or 2 hours after taking an antacid.

53. _____ Watch for injection site reactions.

54. _____ Can cause hypotension.

55. _____ May cause peripheral neuropathy.

56. _____ Report jaundice as drug can cause liver toxicity.

57. _____ Report cough and fever as drug can cause pneumonia.

Categories

A. Nucleoside reverse transcriptase inhibitors
B. Nonnucleoside reverse transcriptase inhibitors
C. Protease inhibitors
D. Integrase inhibitors
E. Fusion inhibitors
F. Entry inhibitors

TEACHING PATIENTS AND FAMILIES ABOUT RETROANTIVIRALS

Fill in the blank for each of the topics below that describe the type of information patients and their families need to be aware of when taking retroantiviral drugs.

58. Take the drugs exactly as ordered every day to ensure the drugs work properly and your disease does not become

    _____ to the drugs.

59. Take the drugs at the same _____ every day and use a cell-phone reminder for time alerts. This way drug levels remain steady, and viral suppression is ideal.

60. Alert your healthcare provider immediately to specific symptoms that may indicate _____ reactions.

61. Safer _____ practice and standard precautions must be taken to prevent disease transmission.

62. Impaired immunity makes it more likely to contract diseases. Avoid eating raw _____ and fish, as well as fruits and vegetables that cannot be peeled or scrubbed.

63. If you are lactating, stop _____ your baby because there is a high risk of HIV transmission in breast milk.

64. Report any new over-the-counter (OTC) drugs, herbs, or _____, illegal drugs, and nutritional supplements to your prescriber because they could cause increased adverse reactions.

65. Avoid alcohol and recreational drugs because of the increased risk for _____ damage associated with these drugs.

66. Report signs of _____: numbness or tingling in feet or hands, which spreads to legs and arms; sharp, jabbing, throbbing, or burning pain in arms and legs; and decreased coordination and falling.

67. If you have symptoms of _____ (upper abdominal pain that may radiate to your back, pain that worsens after eating, increased nausea and vomiting), notify your healthcare provider immediately so treatment can begin early.

PRACTICE QUIZ

1. Which of the following statements most accurately states the purpose of both antiviral and antiretroviral drugs?
   a. If started at the earliest onset of the infection, these drugs can cure the patient who has a virus or retrovirus.
   b. Because of the many side effects and adverse reactions, most healthcare providers are reluctant to prescribe these drugs.
   c. Patients who have been treated with antiviral or antiretroviral drugs once, cannot continue if a second outbreak occurs.
   d. Antiviral and antiretroviral drugs limit or slow the advance of the virus or retrovirus but do not cure the patient.

2. What does combination antiretroviral therapy, or cART, indicate for a patient?
   a. Several types of antiretroviral drugs are used together daily for patients infected by HIV.
   b. Different antiretroviral drugs are given each day of the week, and then the routine is repeated the following week.
   c. This method is used for individuals who are at a high risk for HIV infection.
   d. The combination antiretroviral therapy, or cART, is utilized to prevent attachment of the HIV retrovirus to the outside of the CD4 cell.

3. Which of the following groups of individuals are at the lowest risk for developing HIV infection?
   a. Transgender women who have sex with men
   b. Women who are white and have sex with other women
   c. Minority heterosexual women
   d. Intravenous drug users

4. Which category of antiretroviral drug is given early in the life cycle of an HIV infection?
   a. Protease inhibitors
   b. Fusion inhibitors
   c. Nucleoside reverse transcriptase inhibitors
   d. Entry inhibitors

5. Who is eligible to receive Pre-exposure Prophylaxis (PrEP) drug therapy?
   a. Persons who had sex with an individual who is in the early stages of HIV infection
   b. Healthcare personnel who work extensively with patients who are HIV positive
   c. Sex partners of persons who are HIV positive and using cART
   d. Men who regularly have sex with other men

6. One of the adverse reactions to antivirals and antiretroviral drug therapy is pancreatitis. What is one of the signs or symptoms of pancreatitis?
   a. Upper abdominal pain or pain that radiates to your back
   b. Pain that lessens after eating
   c. Abnormally slow pulse and blood pressure
   d. Jaundiced skin

7. In the United States and Canada, what is one of the most common ways Hepatitis B and Hepatitis C are transmitted?
   a. Contaminated water
   b. Sexual activity
   c. Spoiled meat
   d. Respiratory infections

8. Although the cost is prohibitive for most individuals, what new drug may represent a cure for Hepatitis C?
   a. Harvoni
   b. Virazole
   c. Hepsera
   d. Interferon

9. What are the only two antivirals approved for treating or preventing influenza in children? (Select two.)
   a. Rapivab
   b. Relenza
   c. Amantadine
   d. Tamiflu

10. There are seven steps in the HIV life cycle. At one step, HIV changes the CD4 cell's DNA and the RNA messenger, and the CD4 cell starts making long HIV protein chains. What is this step named?
    a. Replication
    b. Budding
    c. Integration
    d. Assembly

11. Why are the six categories of antiretroviral drugs referred to as inhibitors?
    a. They inhibit all other types of viruses and retroviruses from attacking the cells.
    b. They inhibit bodily functions from becoming over-reactive to HIV.
    c. They suppress retroviral reproduction.
    d. They suppress white blood cell production.

12. How long must a patient continue combination antiretroviral drug therapy (cART)?
    a. Until the CD4 cell counts return to normal
    b. For about 35 years
    c. For the remainder of his or her life
    d. Until the budding phase of the life cycle is complete

13. During pregnancy, which categories of antiretroviral drugs are commonly given to women who are HIV positive? (Select three.)
    a. Nucleoside reverse transcriptase inhibitors
    b. Nonnucleoside reverse transcriptase inhibitors
    c. Protease inhibitors
    d. Entry inhibitors
    e. Fusion inhibitors
    f. Integrase inhibitors

14. What is a sign indicating that the person who was HIV positive has developed full-blown AIDS?
    a. There is an increased number of CD4 cells in the body.
    b. The person develops allergic reactions to the antiretroviral drug therapy.
    c. There is a breakdown in the immune system in which the person is no longer able to fight any infection.
    d. The person is diagnosed with cancers such as pancreatic cancer.

15. Which virus is the common cause of chest colds, croup, and pneumonia in children?
    a. Influenza
    b. RSV
    c. CMV
    d. HPB

7 Drugs for Allergy and Respiratory Problems

IDENTIFYING TYPES OF DRUGS

Match the drug name with the category of drugs.

Drug Names

1. _____ Albuterol

2. _____ Benzonatate

3. _____ Montelukast

4. _____ Guaifenesin

5. _____ Brompheniramine

6. _____ Fexofenadine

7. _____ Fluticasone

8. _____ Promethazine and codeine

9. _____ Ipratropium

10. _____ Zafirlukast

11. _____ Tiotropium

12. _____ Triamcinolone

13. _____ Arformoterol

14. _____ Levalbuterol

15. _____ Formoterol

Drug Categories

A. Antihistamines
B. Leukotriene inhibitors
C. Decongestants
D. Short-acting beta2 agonists
E. Long-acting beta2 agonists
F. Cholinergic antagonists
G. Mucolytics
H. Antitussives

IDENTIFY THE CONDITION

For each of the following scenarios, identify what problem most likely describes what the patient is experiencing.

16. Throughout the week, a newly admitted resident to a rehabilitation center experiences shortness of breath and has a dry hacking cough. These incidents seem to occur every 3 to 4 days.

    _____

17. A patient who is recovering from bilateral knee replacement receives a bouquet of fragrant, blooming flowers. She immediately starts sneezing, and her eyes begin to run.

    _____

18. Your patient seems to continually suffer from a chronic cough that produces clear, white, yellow or green sticky mucus, wheezing, shortness of breath, and complains of chest tightness.

    _____

29

Copyright © 2019, Elsevier Inc. All rights reserved.

Chapter **7 Drugs for Allergy and Respiratory Problems**

FILL IN THE BLANK

19. _____ occurs when the immune system develops a response to an environmental substance that it views as dangerous to the body.

20. _____ is a long-term condition of the airways that causes muscle constriction and inflammation of the airways and lungs. Symptoms are intermittent.

21. _____ is a progressive disease that obstructs airflow passages in the upper and lower airways. Constant inflammation produces large amounts of sticky mucous.

SELECT ALL THAT APPLY

For each of the drug types listed below, check all the statements that are applicable.

22. Antihistamines

_____ Could cause blindness

_____ Increase airflow through the bronchial tubes

_____ Reduce symptoms of sneezing, itching, and runny nose

_____ Could cause increased blood pressure

_____ Could cause slight nosebleed

_____ Drowsiness is an expected side effect.

23. Leukotriene inhibitors

_____ Block histamines to prevent inflammation

_____ Decrease the thickness of respiratory secretions and aid in their removal

_____ Long-term use could lead to liver dysfunction.

_____ Used to reduce symptoms of allergies and asthma

24. Decongestants

_____ Reduce the swelling of nasal passages

_____ Used to relieve or suppress coughing

_____ Overuse can cause insomnia.

_____ Can be used daily for extended periods of time

25. Short-acting beta$_2$-adrenergic agonists (SABAs)

_____ Relax smooth muscles almost immediately

_____ Effects wear off quickly.

_____ Common side effects include depression.

_____ May cause tremors

26. Long-acting beta2-adrenergic agonists

_____ May cause rising intraocular pressure

_____ Taken daily to prevent bronchospasms

_____ Are orally inhaled and bind to beta2-adrenergic receptors

_____ Dry mouth and bad taste are common side effects.

27. Cholinergic antagonists

_____ Are orally inhaled controller drugs

_____ Relax the muscles around the airways

_____ Allow more of the body's own adrenalin to activate beta2 receptors

_____ May cause constipation

28. Mucolytics

_____ Shrink swollen nasal membranes

_____ May cause fungal infection in the nose or throat

_____ Prevent bronchoconstriction in asthma

_____ Decrease the thickness of respiratory secretions and aids in their removal

29. Antitussives

_____ Relieve or suppress coughing

_____ Can work by peripherally anesthetizing stretch receptors in the respiratory tract

_____ Capsules that are not swallowed whole can anesthetize the throat.

_____ Prevent mast and white blood cells from releasing mediators of inflammation

FILL IN THE BLANKS

For the following teaching information for each drug type, fill in the blank(s) with the appropriate word(s).

Antihistamines

30. Unless you must restrict your _____ intake because of another health problem, drink extra _____s to help prevent respiratory tract dryness.

31. Do not drink _____ while taking antihistamines because the CNS depressant effects of antihistamines may be increased.

32. Avoid _____ until you know how antihistamines affect you because they cause drowsiness in many patients.

33. If the drug causes _____ upset, take it with meals or milk to decrease this problem.

Leukotriene inhibitors

34. Report any increase in _____ attacks or allergic symptoms to your healthcare provider.

35. Consider not taking these drugs if you are _____ or breast-feeding.

36. Because these drugs are used to prevent (rather than stop) _____ attacks or allergic responses, do not suddenly stop the drug or decrease doses.

Decongestants

37. Do not use sympathomimetic nasal _____ for more than 3 days because a rebound stuffiness and congestion are likely to occur.

38. If you have high blood pressure or heart problems, check with the pharmacist before using _____-____-_____ cold preparations.

39. If you have _____ or cataracts, check with your healthcare provider before using corticosteroid nasal sprays.

40. Contact your healthcare provider if _____ patches develop in the nose or mouth while taking corticosteroid nasal sprays.

Beta-adrenergic agonists and anticholinergic antagonists

41. Contact your healthcare provider if bronchial _____, dizziness, chest pain, insomnia, or any changes in symptoms occur.

42. Drinking lots of fluid, especially water, makes the _____ thinner and helps the drug work better.

43. To prevent _____-induced bronchospasm, use your reliever bronchodilator inhaler 15 to 30 minutes before starting to _____.

44. After using your inhaler, rinse your mouth with _____ to decrease dry mouth and bad taste.

Mucolytic and antitussive drugs

45. Use a _____ and drink at least 2 quarts of water daily while taking a mucolytic unless there is a medical reason for fluid restriction. These actions will help get the mucus out.

46. Notify your healthcare provider if the cough is present with a high _____, rash, or persistent headaches, or if the cough returns once it has been under control.

47. Take the drug with at least one full glass of _____.

48. Do not take opioid antitussives with _____ or any other drugs that slow the central nervous system because the side effects will be intensified.

MATCHING

Indicate whether each of the steps below is referring to use of (a) metered dose inhaler, (b) dry powder inhaler, or (c) both.

49. _____ Insert the mouthpiece of the inhaler into the nonmouthpiece end of the spacer.

50. _____ Turn the device to the next dose of drug.

51. _____ Fully exhale and then place the mouthpiece into your mouth, over your tongue.

52. _____ Never exhale (breathe out) into your inhaler.

53. _____ Never shake your inhaler.

54. _____ Breathe in slowly and deeply.

55. _____ Never wash or place the inhaler in water.

56. _____ Remove the mouthpiece from your mouth; keeping your lips closed, hold your breath for at least 10 seconds and then breathe out slowly.

57. _____ Place your lips over the mouthpiece and breathe in forcefully. (There is no propellant in the inhaler; only your breath pulls the drug in.)

58. _____ Wait at least 1 minute between puffs.

59. _____ At least once a day, clean the case and cap of the inhaler.

60. _____ Exhale fully away from the inhaler.

PRACTICE QUIZ

1. Which of the following are considered harmless substances that can cause allergic reactions to people who are overly sensitive to them?
   a. Sand and dirt
   b. Dust mites
   c. Concrete parking lots
   d. Iron fences

2. Allergic reactions usually occur at the point of contact with the allergen. If the skin reacts to an allergen and becomes red and/or swollen, what is one common method of drug administration that can be used to lessen the reaction?
   a. Nasal spray
   b. Lung inhalation
   c. Topical cream
   d. Suppository

3. There are two types of histamines, H1 and H2. Antihistamines that block H1 receptors limit bronchoconstriction. What do antihistamines block when focused on H2 receptors?
   a. Skin irritation
   b. Lymph nodes
   c. Stomach acid production
   d. Nasal passage swelling

4. How can an individual procure first-generation antihistamines?
   a. With a prescription from an allergy specialist
   b. Can be purchased over-the-counter
   c. Are available over the Internet from Canada or India
   d. These drugs are no longer produced.

5. When assessing patients before giving antihistamines, what specific information should you obtain?
   a. Determine whether the patient is actually allergic to the substance.
   b. Examine the patient's ears and throat to determine how badly they are affected from the allergic reaction.
   c. Ask whether the patient has objections due to religious reasons for taking any kind of drug.
   d. Ask whether the patient suffers from thyroid disease or migraine headaches.

6. When should leukotriene inhibitors **NOT** be given?
   a. If the patient is having an acute asthma attack
   b. When the patient is not having an acute asthma attack
   c. If a patient has never had asthma
   d. If adults with asthma weigh over 100 pounds

7. How do cromones reduce symptoms of patients with allergies or asthma?
   a. Block leukotriene response
   b. Activate mast cells that control the immune system
   c. Prevent mast cells from opening
   d. Prevent allergic responses to dander

8. What is the function of sympathomimetic drugs?
   a. Mimic stimulation of sympathetic nervous system and shrink blood vessels so the nose can drain more efficiently
   b. Block the body's adrenalin to reduce inflammation in the nasal passages
   c. Slow the production of histamine and leukotriene
   d. Reduce discomfort of skin allergies

9. Which of the following conditions does **NOT** prohibit use of oral sympathomimetic drugs?
   a. High blood pressure
   b. HIV
   c. Sinus infection
   d. Nasal inflammation

10. Why do patients with asthma usually require more than one type of drug to manage the symptoms?
    a. Many drugs become ineffective after long-term usage.
    b. Inflammation narrows airways from the inside, and bronchoconstriction narrows airways from the outside.
    c. Asthma attacks are initiated by allergens, and multiple drugs are necessary to focus on specific allergic reactions.
    d. Asthma has multiple symptoms (e.g., shortness of breath, wheezing, cough).

11. What is one of the usual causes of chronic obstructive pulmonary disease (COPD)?
    a. Allergies to dust mites
    b. Pneumonia
    c. Cigarette smoking
    d. Repeated bouts of bronchitis

12. Drug therapy for both asthma and COPD includes two types of agents. One agent is an anti-inflammatory. What is the other type of agent required for treatment?
    a. Bronchodilating
    b. Sympathomimetic
    c. Corticosteroid
    d. Mast cell stabilizer

13. How do mucolytic drugs decrease the thickness of respiratory secretions?
    a. Enabling patients to cough up large quantities of thick mucus
    b. Increasing the amount of fluid in the respiratory tract
    c. Increasing the size of nasal passages to allow for more productive cough
    d. Enabling patients to drain sinuses more efficiently

14. According to the Food and Drug Administration (FDA), mucolytic drugs should not be given to which of the following patients?
    a. Immunocompromised patients
    b. Elderly patients
    c. Young children
    d. Pregnant or breast-feeding women

15. How do nonopioid antitussives reduce the cough reflex?
    a. Anesthetizing stretch receptors in respiratory passages, lungs, and pleura
    b. Acting directly on the cough center in the medulla of the brain
    c. Thinning the secretions to promote ciliary action
    d. Relaxing the muscles around the airway

Chapter **7** **Drugs for Allergy and Respiratory Problems**

8 Drugs Affecting the Renal/Urinary and Cardiovascular Systems

IDENTIFYING DRUGS BY USE

Match the drug name with its use.

Drug Names

1. _____ Hydrochlorothiazide

2. _____ Quinidine

3. _____ Simvastatin

4. _____ Nitroglycerin

5. _____ Trospium chloride

6. _____ Tamsulosin

7. _____ Quinapril

Drug Use

A. Diuretics
B. Benign prostatic hyperplasia
C. Overactive bladder
D. HMG-CoA reductase inhibitors (statins)
E. Antihypertensive
F. Antianginal
G. Antidysrhythmic

DRUG CATEGORIES

Match the description with each of the drug categories.

Description

8. _____ Slows the conduction of impulses through the heart

9. _____ Relaxes smooth muscle tissue in the prostate gland, the neck of the bladder, and the urethra by binding to the alpha-1 adrenergic receptors, placing less pressure on the urethra and improving urine flow

10. _____ Lowers blood LDL levels by slowing liver production of cholesterol

11. _____ Lowers blood pressure by increasing urine output and preventing water, sodium, potassium, and chloride from being reabsorbed back into the blood

12. _____ Decreases blood pressure by relaxing vascular smooth muscle in the coronary and systemic arteries, leading to decreased peripheral resistance

13. _____ Increases oxygen to the heart, enabling it to pump more easily

14. _____ Inhibits involuntary nerve-induced contractions of the detrusor muscle, relaxing bladder and holding more urine

Drug Categories

A. Thiazides
B. Selective alpha-1 blockers
C. Urinary antispasmodics
D. HMG-CoA reductase inhibitors (statins)
E. Calcium channel blockers
F. Nitrates
G. Sodium channel blockers

IDENTIFYING SIDE/ADVERSE EFFECTS

15. Which of the following are side effects and/or adverse effects of diuretic drugs? Check all that apply.
   a. _____ Urinary urgency and urinary frequency
   b. _____ Flare-ups of gout
   c. _____ Low magnesium
   d. _____ Dehydration

16. Which of the following are side effects and/or adverse effects of HMG-CoA reductase inhibitors (statins)? Check all that apply.
   a. _____ Acid reflux
   b. _____ Sore throat
   c. _____ Jaundice
   d. _____ Muscle breakdown

34

17. Which of the following are side effects and/or adverse effects of nonstatin antihyperlipidemic drugs? Check all that apply.
    a. _____ Gemfibrozil and fenofibrate can cause kidney failure and *cholelithiasis* (gallstones).
    b. _____ Bile acid sequestrants increase absorption of fat-soluble vitamins (A, D, E, and K).
    c. _____ Niacin use can cause *flushing* (red color in the face and neck).
    d. _____ Bile acid sequestrants can cause blood clotting.

18. Which of the following are side effects and/or adverse effects of antihypertensive drugs? Check all that apply.
    a. _____ Calcium channel blockers also work as diuretics.
    b. _____ Beta blockers can cause bronchoconstriction, which is a problem for patients with asthma.
    c. _____ Most antihypertensive drugs can cause dizziness when the patient changes positions.
    d. _____ Patients may experience a dramatic drop in blood pressure.

19. Which of the following are side effects and/or adverse effects of nitrates? Check all that apply.
    a. _____ Throbbing headaches caused by rapid blood-vessel dilation in the head
    b. _____ Severe postural hypertension when a person suddenly stands up
    c. _____ Reflex tachycardia (rapid heartbeat) or paradoxical bradycardia
    d. _____ Vitamin B deficiency

20. Which of the following are side effects and/or adverse effects of inotropic drugs? Check all that apply.
    a. _____ These drugs can produce toxins within the body.
    b. _____ Symptoms of toxins include allergic reactions to nuts and dairy.
    c. _____ Early signs of toxins in infants and the elderly include an unusually rapid heartbeat.
    d. _____ Children often experience hyperactivity and euphoria.

DESCRIBE PATIENT AND FAMILY TEACHING

For each of the following drug types, follow the example provided and list at least three items you should teach patients and families regarding drug use.

21. Diuretics
    ■ Take the drug exactly as prescribed. Do not skip or double doses.
    Your responses

22. HMG-CoA Reductase Inhibitors (Statins)
    ■ Lifestyle changes such as exercise, a low-cholesterol diet, and good weight management are just as important while you are taking the statins to help prevent cardiovascular disease.
    Your responses

23. Niacin or Nicotinic Acid
    ■ Take the drug at the time prescribed because timing is important for cholesterol-lowering drugs.
    Your responses

24. Antihypertensive Drugs
   - Take this drug exactly as ordered. If a dose is missed, it should be taken as soon as it is remembered; if it is close to the next scheduled dose, skip the missed dose and return to the regular dosing schedule.
   Your responses

25. Antianginals
   - Keep the nitroglycerin (NTG) tablets in a dark, glass container to prevent breakdown of the drug.
   Your responses

26. Antidysrhythmics
   - Take this drug exactly as ordered and do not skip doses or double the dose.
   Your responses

27. Inotropic Drugs
   - Let your healthcare provider know if you have any loss of appetite, nausea, vomiting, diarrhea, or any vision changes that can be an indication of digoxin toxicity.
   Your responses

PRACTICE QUIZ

1. How does the renal/urinary system work with the cardiovascular system to maintain adequate circulation in the body?
   a. The two systems ensure the bowels work efficiently.
   b. The two systems help maintain fluid balance.
   c. The two systems regulate heartbeat.
   d. The two systems regulate what comes into the kidney.

2. Your elderly patient is taking a diuretic. What side effects do you need to watch for other than dehydration?
   a. Signs of low potassium
   b. Unusually dry skin
   c. Magnesium deficiency
   d. Change in urine color

3. What symptoms are controlled by phenazopyridine?
   a. Cures urinary tract infection
   b. Treats infections causing irritation to the bladder
   c. Manages color of the urine
   d. Controls burning and pain of the urinary tract

4. Which of the following conditions can cause ischemia?
   a. Dehydration due to overuse of diuretics
   b. Decreased blood flow through the coronary arteries
   c. Decreased kidney output
   d. Increased blood flow through the coronary arteries

5. How is heart failure usually managed in order to reduce associated symptoms?
   a. Depending on other health conditions, patient is put on list for transplant.
   b. Patients increase heart function through diet and exercise.
   c. Patients are given a variety of cardiovascular drugs.
   d. Patients are given antibiotics to ensure optimum systemic health.

36

6. Why should grapefruit juice not be used when a patient is given statins?
   a. Increases liver toxicity
   b. Increases concentration in blood, promoting toxic side effect
   c. Decreases the effectiveness of statins, resulting in poor performance
   d. Causes anaphylactic shock in some patients

7. How does ezetimibe lower cholesterol?
   a. Limits the absorption of cholesterol from food or other sources
   b. Destroys cholesterol cells attached to the intestinal wall
   c. Blocks cholesterol from entering the cardiac system
   d. Limits the ability of cholesterol cells to reproduce within the body

8. The Joint National Committee on the Prevention, Detection, Evaluation, and Treatment of High Blood Pressure recommends best practices for hypertension management. Before beginning drug therapy, what does the Commission recommend as the first attempt in reducing hypertension?
   a. Stress reduction
   b. Vitamin supplements
   c. Surgical intervention
   d. Lifestyle modification

9. Before teaching a patient about possible changes he or she can make to reduce high blood pressure, you need to assess modifiable and nonmodifiable risk factors. Which of the following is a nonmodifiable risk factor?
   a. Smoking
   b. Levels of physical activity
   c. Race
   d. Diet

10. What is the usual cause of a myocardial infarction?
    a. Comorbidities such as renal failure
    b. Rapid heartbeat on a daily basis
    c. Reduction of blood flow to the heart muscle
    d. Niacin deficiency

11. You should not give nitroglycerin if your patient's blood pressure goes below which of the following readings?
    a. 90/60
    b. 110/60
    c. 120/65
    d. 100/70

12. Which term is used to describe irregular heartbeat rhythm?
    a. Arrhythmia
    b. Dysrhythmia
    c. Angithythmia
    d. Cardiothythmia

13. When assessing patients prior to giving digoxin, what is one of the conditions you need to manage?
    a. Ensure the patient is getting sufficient oxygen to the bloodstream.
    b. Ensure the patient's heart rate is 59 or below.
    c. Ensure the patient's heart rate is 60 or above.
    d. Ensure that patient's magnesium level is normal.

14. How can you monitor a nursing-home patient who is taking diuretics to ensure he doesn't become dehydrated?
    a. Weigh the patient on a daily basis.
    b. Test the skin for flexibility.
    c. Ensure the patient drinks 64 ounces of water per day.
    d. Record each time the patient urinates and monitor the amount.

15. Should statins be given in the evening or in the morning?
    a. All statins should be given in the morning.
    b. It does not matter at what time of day statins are given as long as it is done consistently.
    c. It varies by the type of drug prescribed.
    d. It is preferable to give statins at bedtime.

9 Drug Therapy for Central Nervous System Problems

DRUGS FOR PARKINSON DISEASE

FILL IN THE BLANKS

1. Parkinson disease is a disorder of the central nervous system and indicates a lack of _____.

2. Without dopamine, movements become hard to control and some muscles are _____.

3. Arms and legs "catch" at certain points in a "stop-and-go" fashion known as _____ rigidity.

4. Other symptoms include "mask-like" facial features, risk for falls, tremors, and difficulty chewing, swallowing, and _____.

5. Frequent complications include _____, hallucinations, and anxiety.

MATCHING

Match the items on the left, which include related drug information (names, descriptions, and administration details), with the Parkinson disease drug types on the right. You will use each drug type more than once.

Drug Information

6. _____ Entacapone

7. _____ Safinamide

8. _____ Increases dopamine levels of the brain

9. _____ Patients should avoid foods and beverages containing large amounts of tyramine.

10. _____ Carbidopa/levodopa tablets

11. _____ High-protein foods decrease absorption.

12. _____ Allows existing dopamine to remain active in the brain longer

13. _____ Pramipexo

14. _____ Helps dopamine and dopamine-agonist drugs to remain active in the body longer

15. _____ Give 30–60 minutes before meals

16. _____ May turn urine to orange-brown color

17. _____ Rasagiline

18. _____ Give these drugs at the same time every day.

19. _____ Tolcapone

20. _____ Sinemet

Drug Types

A. Dopamine agonists
B. Catechol-O-methyltransferase (COMT) inhibitors
C. Selective monoamine oxidase B (MAO-B) inhibitors

TRUE OR FALSE

Indicate True (T) or False (F) for each of the following statements regarding side effects/adverse reactions to drugs that treat the symptoms of Parkinson disease.

21. _____ One of the most common side effects of carbidopa/levodopa and all dopamine agonists is the eruption of cold sores around the mouth.

22. _____ The most common adverse reaction to Rytary is dyskinesia.

23. _____ If a patient is taking dopamine agonists and suffers from delirium, psychosis, or hallucinations, this is related to the disease process not from the drug.

24. _____ As carbidopa/levodopa dosages are decreased as COMT inhibitors and MAO-B inhibitors are added to the drug regime, the patient could experience neuroleptic malignant syndrome.

25. _____ The effectiveness of dopamine agonists is reduced when taken with a steak dinner.

SHORT ANSWER

26. When is the best time to give dopamine agonists in conjunction with meals or snacks?

27. If the patient is taking levodopa, which vitamin is contraindicated because it accelerates the inactivation of the drug?

28. About how soon will you begin to see clinical improvements in a patient who begins taking drugs that treat the symptoms of Parkinson disease?

29. When taking MAO-B inhibitors, what are some of the symptoms, which if suddenly worsen, indicate you should contact the healthcare provider immediately?

30. What instructions should you give to your patients to help them avoid falling due to low blood pressure, which can result from drugs used to treat the symptoms of Parkinson disease?

DRUGS FOR ALZHEIMER DISEASE

FILL IN THE BLANK

1. Alzheimer disease is one of many forms of _____, which is the progressive loss of brain function.

2. Alzheimer disease causes changes to multiple aspects of the brain; over time, these changes _____ the size of the brain and all aspects of brain function.

3. Drugs, which include cholinesterase inhibitors and NMDA blockers, provide _____ improvement in symptoms.

4. Symptoms of Alzheimer disease begin with memory issues, which get progressively worse and eventually include confusion, as well as changes in mood, judgment, and _____.

5. When evaluating a patient for Alzheimer disease, it is important to know the risk factors, which include age greater than 65, family history, and having the APOE-e4 _____.

MATCHING

Match the items on the left, which include related drug information (names, descriptions, and administration details), with the Alzheimer disease drug types on the right. You will use each drug type more than once.

Drug Information

6. _____ Binds to acetylcholinesterase enzyme and slows its breakdown of acetylcholine

7. _____ Galantamine

8. _____ Memantine

9. _____ Donepezil

10. _____ Adverse effects include somnolence.

11. _____ Monitor patients taking these drugs for worsening asthma conditions and GI bleeds.

12. _____ Reduces neuronal damage by protecting neurons from calcium

Drug Types

A. Cholinesterase inhibitors
B. NMDA (N-methyl-D-aspartate) blockers

TRUE OR FALSE

Indicate True (T) or False (F) for each of the following statements regarding drugs that treat the symptoms of Alzheimer disease.

13. _____ If Alzheimer disease is diagnosed at an early stage, a combination of cholinesterase inhibitors and NMDA blockers can alleviate the disease entirely.

14. _____ Aricept should be taken at bedtime.

15. _____ Patients taking cholinesterase inhibitors should urinate every 2 hours to prevent incontinence.

16. _____ NMDA blockers that come in extended-release capsules must be taken whole.

17. _____ If using a liquid form of NMDA blocker, it can be mixed with other liquids to improve taste.

18. _____ If a patient is taking NMDA blockers, it is important to monitor the patient's blood pressure.

19. What is one adverse effect applicable to both cholinesterase inhibitors and NMDA blockers?

20. To evaluate a patient for symptom improvement, before he starts a cholinesterase inhibitor, how should you assess him?

21. Why should you assess a patient for swallowing difficulties?

22. Why should patients with risk for renal impairment be cautioned prior to taking memantine?

DRUGS FOR EPILEPSY

FILL IN THE BLANK

1. Epilepsy is a type of chronic _____ disorder in which brain neurons become hyperexcitable and trigger unneeded electrical signals.

2. Seizures are the body's response to those inappropriate _____ signals.

3. A _____ is the sudden contraction of many muscle groups without the person's conscious control.

4. Based on symptoms, length, and degree of consciousness, seizures are classified first as _____ or generalized.

TRUE OR FALSE

Indicate True (T) or False (F) for each of the following statements regarding drugs that treat the symptoms of epilepsy.

5. _____ Phenytoin can be used safely with patients who are pregnant.

6. _____ Carbamazepine use increases a patient's risk of sunburn.

7. _____ Phenobarbital can cause depression of the central nervous system.

8. _____ Valproic acid is not recommended for patients who are diagnosed with COPD due to the possibility of depression of the respiratory system.

9. _____ Amnesia is a potential adverse reaction to lamotrigine.

10. _____ Lacosamide has been known to cause euphoria in patients and is therefore sometimes given as an antidepressant.

11. _____ Topiramine use is associated with memory loss.

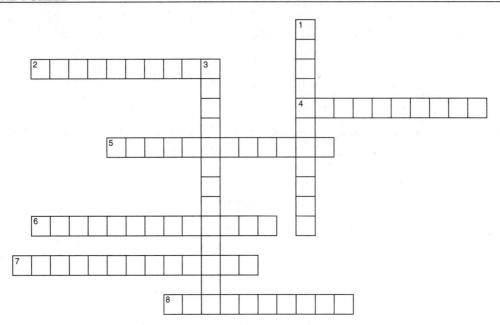

Across

2. Appears to stabilize neuron membranes and prevent repetitive excitation and firing
4. Appears to reduce seizures by preventing spread of excitation in brain GABA
5. Increases the activity of the inhibitory neurotransmitter GABA
6. Enhances the action of the inhibitory neurotransmitter
7. Limits spread of neuron excitation by altering the sodium channels of nerve membranes
8. Prevents spread of neuron excitation binding to sodium channels on nerve membranes

Down

1. Unknown action thought to reduce seizures by blocking sodium channels on neuron membranes
3. Reduces seizures by altering calcium channels on the neuron membrane

Word Banks: CARBAMAZEPINE, EUTHOSUXIMIDE, LACOSAMIDE, LAMOTRIGINE, PHENOBARBITAL, PHENYTOINS, TOPIRAMINE, VALPROICACID

MATCHING

Match the patient teaching descriptions on the left with the epilepsy drug on the right. You may use each drug type more than once.

Teaching Descriptions

Drugs

12. _____ Warn patient to note symptoms of metabolic acidosis such as slow heart rate and warm flushed skin.

13. _____ Can cause bradycardia so take pulse daily and report changes and irregularities.

14. _____ Check daily for rashes.

15. _____ Ask provider if folic acid supplements are needed.

16. _____ Increased risk of falls

17. _____ Can cause tachycardia so take pulse daily and report changes and irregularities.

18. _____ Do not increase dosage to improve mood-enhancing properties.

19. _____ Take with meals to avoid GI distress.

20. _____ Use good oral hygiene to prevent gum disease.

21. _____ Note changes in respiratory functions.

22. _____ Parents should observe children for signs of yellowing skin.

23. _____ Report headaches and muscle weakness, which could be signs of low sodium.

24. _____ Warn patient to note symptoms of encephalopathy such as lethargy or vomiting.

25. _____ May be used when pregnant

A. Phenytoins
B. Carbamazepine
C. Euthosuximide
D. Phenobarbital
E. Valproic acid
F. Oxcarbazepine
G. Lamotrigine
H. Lacosamide
I. Topiramine

DRUGS FOR MULTIPLE SCLEROSIS

FILL IN THE BLANK

1. Multiple sclerosis (MS) is an autoimmune disease affecting the _____ in the brain and spinal cord.

2. Symptoms of multiple sclerosis occur when the nerve transmission is _____.

3. Multiple sclerosis is more common in _____ than _____.

4. Multiple sclerosis cannot be cured, but drug therapy can slow _____.

5. In the past, there were no specific drugs for treatment of MS; therefore patient drug therapy consisted of anti-inflammatories, such as _____.

6. Biologic response modifiers modify the patient's immune response to abnormal _____ for immunity and inflammation.

7. Monoclonal antibodies for MS attack and either inactivate or destroy _____ that damage the myelin.

8. Neurologic drugs for MS either protect nerves and myelin from destruction or improve impulse _____ of demyelinated nerves.

MATCHING

Match the drugs for relapsing-remitting multiple sclerosis on the left with the drug types on the right. You may use each drug type more than once.

Drug Names

9. _____ Dimethyl fumarate

10. _____ Beta-interferon

11. _____ Ocrelizumab

12. _____ Dalfampridine

13. _____ Alemtuzumab

14. _____ Fingolimod

Drug Types

A. Biologic response modifiers
B. Monoclonal antibodies
C. Neurologic drugs

SYMPTOMS

Select which of the symptoms are associated with each of the multiple sclerosis drug types.

15. Biologic response modifiers
- ☐ Earache
- ☐ Peripheral neuropathy
- ☐ Increased urinary tract infections (UTIs)
- ☐ Slow heart rate
- ☐ Thinning scalp hair

16. Monoclonal antibodies
- ☐ Increased risk for infection
- ☐ Higher risk for pneumonia
- ☐ Foot pain
- ☐ Hypertension
- ☐ Edema

17. Neurologic drugs
- ☐ Headache, dizziness, muscle weakness
- ☐ GI problems, heartburn, constipation
- ☐ Confusion, seizure activity
- ☐ Nausea, diarrhea, abdominal pain
- ☐ Flushing, itching, rashes

PRACTICE QUIZ

1. What is the composition of the central nervous system?
   a. Nerves extending from the spinal cord
   b. Organs, limbs, muscles, and blood vessels
   c. Brain and spinal cord
   d. Brain, heart, liver, lungs, and kidneys

2. What are the chemicals released from nerve endings that bind with subsequent nerves?
   a. Neurotransmitters
   b. Myelin
   c. Enzymes
   d. Epinephrine

3. The reduction of what chemical within the central nervous system causes Parkinson disease?
   a. Substantia nigra
   b. Acetylcholine
   c. Dopamine
   d. Serotonin

4. When a patient diagnosed with Parkinson disease develops cogwheel rigidity, what is the implication for the patient's movement?
   a. Facial features become mask-like.
   b. Arms and legs catch in stop-and-go movement.
   c. Muscles become overly relaxed.
   d. Hand tremors are present.

5. Why will all patients with Parkinson disease eventually require dopamine?
   a. All other drug therapies wear off after age 70.
   b. It is converted to natural dopamine.
   c. It reduces overproduction of dopamine caused by other drug therapies.
   d. It reduces symptoms of dyskinesia.

6. At what point are cholinesterase inhibitors no longer effective in the treatment of Alzheimer disease?
   a. When the brain size shrinks and can no longer produce acetylcholinesterase
   b. When the number of neural transmitters sufficiently decreases
   c. When the patient's ability to swallow is impaired
   d. When there are fewer intact neurons available to make acetylcholine

7. What kinds of patient information does the Alzheimer Disease Assessment Scale evaluate?
   a. Multiple organ functions
   b. Cognition, behavior, quality of life
   c. Chemical production within the central nervous system
   d. Muscle and respiratory fitness

8. Although antiepileptic drugs can reduce or prevent seizures, what is another use?
   a. They can be used temporarily to reduce anxiety.
   b. They can be used to fight certain types of neural infections.
   c. They can be used to reduce muscle fatigue in patients with Parkinson disease.
   d. They can be used to increase brain activity in patients with late-stage Alzheimer disease.

9. Most of the newer antiepileptic drugs are used along with other drugs, which is referred to as what kind of drug therapy?
   a. Monotherapy
   b. Adjuvant therapy
   c. Multi-agent neurotherapy
   d. Antigen therapy

10. What is one of the side effects that is common to many of the antiepileptic drugs?
    a. Rash
    b. Increased sodium levels
    c. Folic acid deficiency
    d. Blurred or double vision

11. What is the most common form of multiple sclerosis (MS)?
    a. Relapsing-Remitting MS
    b. Secondary-Progressive MS
    c. Primary-Progressive MS
    d. Progressive-Relapsing MS

12. What drug type was originally the only type of drug therapy available for patients with multiple sclerosis?
    a. Biologic response modifiers
    b. Corticosteroids
    c. Monoclonal antibodies
    d. Neurologic drugs

45

Copyright © 2019, Elsevier Inc. All rights reserved.

Chapter **9 Drug Therapy for Central Nervous System Problems**

10 Drug Therapy for Mental Health and Behavioral Problems

MULTIPLE CHOICE

Select the best answer for each of these following questions about mental health.

1. Which of the following is the best definition of mental illness?
   a. Mental illness results from genetic predispositions and drug or alcohol abuse.
   b. Mental illness is a condition that impacts a person's ability to think and also includes changes in behaviors and emotions.
   c. Mental illness is a condition defined by how an individual relates to environmental stressors and whether the behavior exhibited is considered clinically normal.
   d. Mental illness results from traumatic incidents and an individual's inability to process the experience in a mentally healthy way.

2. Along the continuum of mental health or mental illness, which of the following best indicates when an individual is experiencing mental illness?
   a. Experiencing and coping with stress to mild distress
   b. Increased use of food to cope with stress
   c. Mild or temporary impairment due to coping with distress
   d. Moodiness, including tears and/or inappropriate behavior

3. According to the National Institute of Mental Health, about how many adults experience some degree of mental illness?
   a. 22%
   b. 4%
   c. 18% of women and 4% of men
   d. 18%

4. When a patient experiences sleep deprivation over an extended period of time, what are some of the more obvious impairments he or she might exhibit?
   a. Hand trembling, nervous tics
   b. Difficulty with remembering, judgment, coordination
   c. Snoring, nausea, muscle pain
   d. Gregariousness, introversion, talkativeness

5. Which of the following diagnoses is associated with persons who have chronic or disabling anxiety?
   a. Insomnia
   b. Conduct disorder
   c. Attention-deficit disorder
   d. Social anxiety disorder

6. What is a general definition of psychosis?
   a. Loss of contact with reality
   b. Symptoms of delirium lasting more than 90 days
   c. Condition that is diagnosed such as schizophrenia or dementia
   d. Symptoms of delirium induced by alcohol or drugs

7. Which of the following is a common symptom of significant depression?
   a. Sadness triggered by the loss of a loved one
   b. Crying on a daily basis while at home or in the office
   c. Prolonged inability to perform activities of daily living
   d. Loss of interest in sex

8. Mood stabilizers are prescribed primarily for patients with what kind of illness?
   a. Bipolar illness
   b. Schizophrenia
   c. Depression
   d. Delirium

MATCHING

Match the chemical neurotransmitter on the right with the area affected on the left.

Areas Affected by Neurotransmitter

9. _____ Learning, movement, motivation, and drive

10. _____ Parasympathetic nervous system

11. _____ Sympathetic nervous system, alertness, and arousal

12. _____ Sleep, appetite, pain, and mood

13. _____ Inhibitory neurotransmitter, sleep, and muscle tension

Neurotransmitters

A. Norepinephrine
B. Serotonin
C. Dopamine
D. Gamma-aminobutyric acid (GABA)
E. Acetylcholine

SELECT ALL THAT APPLY

For each of the drugs listed below, check all the statements that are true.

14. Benzodiazepines

_____ Used primarily for pregnant women

_____ Sedating-hypnotic drug that depresses the central nervous system

_____ High risk of dependency

_____ Enhance dopamine effects, leading to reduction in anxiety

15. Nonbenzodiazepine

_____ Makes the central nervous system less responsive to stimuli

_____ May be used to reduce anxiety

_____ Safe for use with patients who have liver impairment

16. Buspirone

_____ Reduces anxiety by affecting the serotonin and GABA neurotransmitters

_____ Decreases muscle tension, sweating, and rapid heart rate

_____ Sedation is possible and high risk for physical dependence

17. Typical antipsychotics

_____ Block dopamine receptors to treat symptoms such as hallucinations and delusions

_____ Can create pseudo-Parkinsonism

_____ Side effects include headache and drowsiness.

_____ Adverse reactions can include neuroleptic malignant syndrome that is characterized by an abnormally low body temperature.

18. Atypical antipsychotics

_____ Used primarily for depression and anxiety

_____ May block dopamine receptors as well as some subtypes of serotonin

_____ Recommended for patients with psychosis from dementia

_____ Most common side effects are insomnia and drowsiness.

_____ Clozapine is associated with decreased white blood cell count.

_____ Weight loss is common.

19. Selective serotonin reuptake inhibitors (SSRIs)

_____ Increase concentration of serotonin available to bind to dopamine receptors

_____ Sexual side effects are common in both men and women.

_____ Increased risk of suicide

_____ Adverse effects include low sodium level.

_____ Safe for women who are pregnant or nursing

20. Serotonin norepinephrine reuptake inhibitors (SNRIs)

_____ Increase concentration of serotonin and norepinephrine neurotransmitters available to postsynaptic receptors

_____ Used for depression, fibromyalgia, and diabetic neuropathy

_____ Side effects include increased appetite.

_____ Some patients experience increased sweating.

_____ Adverse effects include nosebleeds.

_____ Some patients can experience low sodium levels.

21. Tricyclic antidepressants (TCAs)

_____ Have more side effects than SSRIs and SNRIs

_____ Reserved for individuals who do not respond to other treatments

_____ Used for patients with obsessive-compulsive disorder

_____ Can cause vision problems

_____ Can cause delirium in older patients with cognitive impairment

22. Monoamine oxidase (MAO) inhibitors

_____ MAOs are enzymes that break down neurotransmitters.

_____ Used to treat eating disorders

_____ Weight loss occurs in almost 10% of patients.

_____ May cause hypotension if the patient ingests aged cheese and other foods and drinks containing tyramine

47

23. Mood stabilizers

_____ Lithium is used in short-term therapy of acute mania.

_____ Lithium does not cause sedation or euphoria.

_____ Lithium can cause mild weight gain.

_____ Hand tremors are frequent.

_____ Adverse reactions include hyperthyroidism.

FILL IN THE BLANK

Patient and Family Education

24. Only take drugs for sleep if you have 5 to 6 hours available in order to avoid excessive _____.

25. Do not take a sedative with _____ or any other drug that depresses the central nervous system.

26. Nonbenzodiazepine drugs can cause you to be _____ active at night.

27. Avoid drinking _____ juice when taking benzodiazepines and nonbenzodiazepines.

28. Effects of drugs can decrease through use of _____ products and _____ beverages.

29. Suddenly stopping typical antipsychotics can result in nausea, dizziness, and _____.

30. Typical antipsychotics can affect your body's ability to adjust to changes in _____.

31. If you develop unusual muscle _____ while taking typical antipsychotics, contact your healthcare provider.

32. You can take most atypical antipsychotics with _____ to avoid GI upset.

33. Take SSRIs in the _____ to avoid insomnia.

34. St. John's Wort can cause adverse effects if taken with _____.

35. Some patients have increased thoughts of _____ when first taking SSRIs and SNRIs.

36. Taking SNRIs during pregnancy can cause _____ abstinence syndrome in newborns.

37. It may take several _____ on SNRIs before you feel better.

38. TCAs can cause you to be more sensitive to _____ so wear protective clothing.

39. When taking TCAs, you should wear a medical alert _____.

40. The effects of MAO inhibitors can still be in your system for up to _____ weeks after discontinuing the drug.

41. Notify your healthcare provider if you experience a sudden _____ while taking MAO inhibitors.

42. You can mix the liquid version of lithium with _____ juices or other flavored drinks.

43. Avoid significant changes in your _____ and fluid intake.

44. Physical exertion can increase _____ and increase risk of lithium levels.

MATCHING

Match the drug on the left with the appropriate drug category on the right.

Drug Names

45. _____ Imipramine

46. _____ Estazolam

47. _____ Fluoxetine

48. _____ Venlafaxine

49. _____ Chlorpromazine

50. _____ Sertoline

51. _____ Aripiprazole

52. _____ Haloperidol

53. _____ Phenelzine

54. _____ Risperidone

55. _____ Zaleplon

56. _____ Lorazepam

57. _____ Lithium

58. _____ Buproprion

59. _____ Duloxetine

Drug Categories

A. Benzodiazepines
B. Nonbenzodiazepines
C. Typical antipsychotics
D. Atypical antipsychotics
E. Dopamine system stabilizers
F. Atypical antidepressants
G. Selective serotonin reuptake inhibitors
H. Serotonin and norepinephrine reuptake inhibitors
I. Tricyclic antidepressants
J. Monoamine oxidase inhibitors
K. Mood stabilizers

PRACTICE QUIZ

1. What is the main purpose of sedatives?
   a. To reduce anxiety in individuals who are unable to function due to stress
   b. To treat bipolar disease and reduce the symptoms that cause individuals to be anxious
   c. To promote sleep by changing signals in the central nervous system and reducing responses to stimulation
   d. To block neurotransmitters that are overactive and lead to hyperactivity in patients who are unable to sleep

2. Why is caffeine not recommended when taking either nonbenzodiazepines or benzodiazepines?
   a. Caffeine reduces the effectiveness of sedative drugs.
   b. Caffeine causes central nervous system depression, which deepens the sedative effect and can lead to death.
   c. Caffeine and sedatives combined can decrease the effectiveness of oral contraceptives.
   d. Caffeine can be used as an antidote for overdoses of sedatives.

3. Which disorder is **NOT** considered an anxiety disorder?
   a. Post-traumatic stress disorder
   b. Obsessive-compulsive disorder
   c. Panic disorder
   d. Bipolar disorder

4. For long-term mental health concerns, what are some of the best nonpharmacological therapies, other than counseling, for which you can provide information to your patient to assist in his or her recovery?
   a. Weight training, pet therapy, volunteering at a homeless shelter
   b. Vacation, spa days, socializing at a friendly tavern
   c. Mindfulness training, meditation, yoga
   d. Vegan diet, reading inspirational books, religious practice

5. Which of the following is a positive symptom of schizophrenia?
   a. Hallucinations
   b. Muscle rigidity
   c. Flat affect
   d. Cessation of delirium

6. Which of the following is a negative symptom of schizophrenia?
   a. Hallucinations
   b. Muscle rigidity
   c. Flat affect
   d. Cessation of delirium

7. What condition significantly contributes to the disease of schizophrenia?
   a. Overstimulation of dopamine
   b. Lack of serotonin
   c. Overstimulation of central nervous system
   d. Lack of norepinephrine

8. What is the main adverse effect to typical antipsychotic drugs?
   a. Drug dependence and possible addiction
   b. Extrapyramidal symptoms related to decrease in dopamine
   c. Greater rate of cognitive impairment and stroke risk
   d. Extreme fatigue due to increase in serotonin

9. While most extrapyramidal symptoms occur several days or weeks after beginning drug therapy, what symptoms can occur after long-term use or even after the drug is discontinued?
   a. Akathesia
   b. Pseudoparkinsonism
   c. Acute dystonia
   d. Tardive dyskinesia

10. What is one of the advantages of taking atypical antipsychotics rather than typical antipsychotics?
    a. The chances of drug dependency are greatly reduced.
    b. They are recommended for patients with psychosis from dementia.
    c. They treat the negative as well as the positive symptoms common in some mental illnesses.
    d. They do not block dopamine receptors.

11. In addition to mental illnesses such as schizophrenia, what other disorders can be treated by dopamine system stabilizers?
    a. Sleep disorders
    b. Parkinson disease
    c. Tourette syndrome
    d. Epilepsy

12. Mild to moderate depression that lasts up to 2 years is labeled as what type of disorder?
    a. Mood disorder
    b. Dysthymic disorder
    c. Bipolar I disorder
    d. Chronic depression disorder

13. Which of the listed items can increase a patient's risk of serotonin syndrome?
    a. St. John's Wort
    b. Typical antipsychotic drugs
    c. NSAIDs
    d. Caffeinated beverages

14. Which foods containing tyramine should not be ingested when a patient is taking monoamine oxidase inhibitors?
    a. Beef, salmon, dairy
    b. Cured or smoked meats, beer, wine, overripe fruits
    c. Foods containing gluten such as breads and pastas
    d. Overly processed foods such as cookies, chips, boxed foods

15. How do mood stabilizers work with patients diagnosed with bipolar disorder?
    a. Prevent the patient from becoming too depressed
    b. Eventually alleviate all symptoms over a period of time when supplemented with talk therapy
    c. Manage symptoms associated with both mania and depression
    d. Reduce the "highs" associated with the disorder to enable patient to function in most environments

11 Drugs for Pain Management

CROSSWORD PUZZLE

Identify the miscellaneous drug based on the type of pain it most commonly relieves.

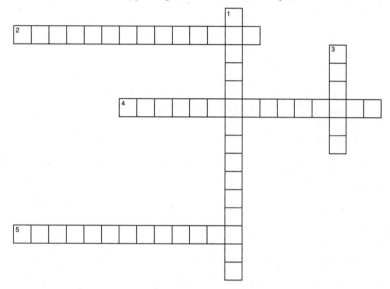

ACROSS

2. Improves long-term sadness and helps manage certain types of chronic pain such as neuropathy
4. Provides powerful anti-inflammatory actions
5. Manages mild to moderate pain and often used in place of aspirin

DOWN

1. Reduces brain seizures and helps minimize pain from neuropathy and migraines
3. Manages pain associated with inflammation, bone pain, cancer pain, and soft-tissue trauma

MATCHING

Match the types of pain management drugs on the left with the drug categories on the right. Each category can be selected more than once.

Pain Management Drugs

6. _____ Fentanyl

7. _____ Tylenol

8. _____ Pentazocine

9. _____ Buprenorphine

10. _____ Clonidine

11. _____ Hydrocodone

12. _____ Aspirin

13. _____ Tramadol

Drug Categories

A. Opioid agonists
B. Opioid agonist-antagonists
C. Nonopioid centrally acting analgesics
D. Miscellaneous analgesics

FILL IN THE BLANK

Identify the type of pain (severe, moderate, mild) most frequently managed with each of the categories.

14. Opiod agonists such as morphine are used most often to manage _____ acute or chronic pain.

15. Opiod agonist-antagonists are used to manage _____ pain, primarily because there is a lower risk for addiction.

16. Nonopiod centrally acting analgesics block pain at the source and can also be used to manage _____ acute pain and lower blood pressure.

17. Miscellaneous analgesics can in some cases be purchased over-the-counter and are used to manage _____ pain. Some forms are able to reduce inflammation.

MATCHING

Match each side effect and/or adverse reaction on the left with the specific type of drug on the right.

Side Effect and/or Adverse Reaction

18. _____ Elevation of blood pressure

19. _____ Increased risk for bleeding

20. _____ Cardiac dysrhythmias

21. _____ Hypotension

22. _____ High dose for prolonged periods can cause liver damage.

23. _____ Sleepiness, constipation, and respiratory depression

24. _____ Blurred vision, dizziness, and urinary retention

25. _____ Seizures

Drug

A. Morphine
B. Pentazocine
C. Buprenorphine
D. Clonidine
E. Tramadol
F. Acetaminophen
G. NSAIDs
H. Cyclobenzaprine

SHORT ANSWERS

Write a brief description of how you would manage each of the following situations.

26. Mrs. Smith has been receiving morphine for several days. What is one question you would ask her to ensure she will not experience further discomfort?

27. Mr. Jones has been given a prescription for an opioid and will be cared for by his wife. You are providing her with information for his care. How can she help prevent dizziness and falling?

28. Ms. Washington has been prescribed tramadol for a back injury. What is an important question to ask her before she begins this drug?

29. After giving Mr. Reyes his first dose of cyclobenzaprine, what should you assess on an hourly basis?

PRACTICE QUIZ

1. How do you assess whether a patient is experiencing pain?
   a. By observing his or her body movements
   b. By asking the patient to identify whether he or she is in pain
   c. Based on when the patient last received a prescribed dosage of pain relief drug
   d. By monitoring vital signs to determine if there are significant changes

2. Identify which of the following situations is likely acute (A) or chronic (C) pain.
   a. _____ Osteoarthritis of the knee
   b. _____ Urinary tract infection
   c. _____ Broken bone
   d. _____ Chemo-induced peripheral neuropathy

3. Which of the following conditions is most likely to increase a patient's perception of pain?
   a. A stroke that destroys a part of the brain
   b. Anxiety and/or depression
   c. A quiet, relaxing environment
   d. Regular use of alternative therapies such as meditation

4. Identify which of the following is not an Agency for Healthcare Research and Quality principle for pain management.
   a. Use of pain intensity scales in order to assess pain systematically
   b. Making sure to ask about pain on a regular basis
   c. Not trusting the patient or family regarding their perceptions or opinions regarding pain
   d. Allowing patients to manage their pain management as much as possible

5. You have a patient still in pain but cannot reach the healthcare provider for a prescription. There are several nondrug options that you can utilize instead. Which of the following, however, would **NOT** be a suitable nondrug therapy for pain relief?
   a. Ice or cold compresses
   b. Six ounces of red wine or 1 ounce of liquor
   c. Exercise
   d. Acupuncture

6. Analgesics are a category of drug developed specifically to reduce pain. How do these drugs work when given to a patient who is in pain?
   a. Change the patient's perception of pain or reduce painful stimulation at its source
   b. Calm the patient to an extent where he or she does not register any pain
   c. Address the source of the actual pain by reducing inflammation
   d. Create a sense of euphoria in the patient so that he or she forgets about the pain

7. Opioids are an analgesic drug used to manage severe pain. Natural opioids are derived from opium. What are synthetic opioids, such as hydrocodone and oxycodone, made from?
   a. Heroin
   b. Morphine
   c. Coca plant
   d. Poppy plant

8. What is the reason all opioids, both natural and synthetic, are labeled *high-alert drugs*?
   a. They must be kept under lock and key to prevent theft because of their cost.
   b. Patients can occasionally become overly excited when taking opioids.
   c. Allergic reactions are frequent with their use.
   d. They have an increased risk for causing patient harm.

Chapter **11 Drugs for Pain Management**

9. Morphine is the drug by which all other pain-management drugs are compared for effectiveness. Which drug from the list below is actually stronger than morphine?
   a. Codeine
   b. Hydrocodone
   c. Delaudid
   d. Oxycodone

10. If a patient taking an opioid agonist, such as morphine, has a strong adverse reaction or overdose, how can the effects be reversed?
    a. Induce vomiting by giving an emetic.
    b. Give an opioid antagonist such as naloxone.
    c. Inject fentanyl intramuscularly or subcutaneously.
    d. Keep the patient awake and help him or her move as much as possible until the effects diminish.

11. Opioid agonist-antagonists are used for less severe pain and are less addictive than opioid agonists but can be responsible for causing which of the following reactions?
    a. Severe cardiac reactions
    b. Severe diarrhea
    c. Severe respiratory reactions
    d. Severe dehydration

12. How do nonopioid centrally acting analgesics, such as clonidine and tramadol, help manage pain?
    a. Interacting with opioid receptors
    b. Stimulating the endorphins
    c. Blocking activity in the central nervous system
    d. Enhancing a feeling of euphoria

13. Which drug can lead to hypotension through dilation of blood vessels?
    a. Tramadol
    b. Butorphanol
    c. Oxycontin
    d. Clonidine

14. Miscellaneous analgesics are used to treat less severe pain and, unlike opioids, can reduce symptoms of pain by which of the following methods?
    a. Increasing the production of endorphins to promote healing
    b. Reducing the symptoms of inflammation by helping stop tissue production of the chemical of inflammation
    c. Raising blood pressure to provide more blood flow to sites that are damaged
    d. Preventing dehydration

15. Which of the following drugs is used to reduce pain from muscular contractions or spasms?
    a. Cyclobenzaprine
    b. Nabumetone
    c. Prednisone
    d. Acetaminophen

12 Anti-inflammatory, Anti-arthritis, and Antigout Drugs

IDENTIFYING TYPES OF DRUGS

Match the drug name with the category of drugs.

Drugs

1. _____ Aspirin
2. _____ Prednisone
3. _____ Etamercept
4. _____ Triamcinolone
5. _____ Nabumetone
6. _____ Meloxicam
7. _____ Allopurinol
8. _____ Celecoxib
9. _____ Adalimumab
10. _____ Dexamethasone

Drug Categories

A. Cyclooxygenase 1 and 2 (COX-1) inhibitors (nonselective NSAIDs)
B. Cyclooxygenase 2 (COX-2) inhibitors (selective NSAIDs)
C. Corticosteroids
D. Disease-modifying antirheumatic drugs
E. Uric acid synthesis inhibitors

SELECT ALL THAT APPLY

Identify all the statements that are applicable for each of the drug categories.

11. Nonsteroidal Anti-inflammatory Drugs (NSAIDs)

_____ Rapidly increase production of one or more inflammatory mediators

_____ COX-1 inhibitor drugs block both COX-1 and COX-2 enzymes when inflammation occurs within the body.

_____ NSAIDs are the first-line therapy against illnesses associated with pain and/or fever.

_____ NSAIDs are not used for any type of arthritis.

_____ Monitor patients who take aspirin for bleeding

Adverse Reactions to NSAIDs

_____ Mild to serious allergic reactions

_____ Severe GI distress

_____ Myocardial infarction and stroke

_____ Reye syndrome in elderly

12. Corticosteroids

_____ Manage severe or chronic inflammation

_____ Used in any condition that could lead to tissue damage

_____ Slow production of red blood cells

_____ Can only be given orally

Adverse Reactions to Corticosteroids

_____ Adrenal glands quit producing cortisol.

_____ Increased number of white blood cells

_____ Delirium or extreme behavior changes

_____ Respiratory failure

13. Disease-modifying Antirheumatic Drugs (DMARDs)

_____ Reduce tissue damage of the inflammatory disease process by inhibiting cortisol

_____ Inhibit inflammatory mediator tumor necrosis factor (TNF)

_____ Tissue damage is reduced but pain is not relieved, so patients require additional drugs to relieve pain and improve physical function.

_____ DMARDs are used in the treatment of chronic inflammatory diseases that involve tissue destruction caused by excessive inflammatory mediators.

Adverse Reactions to DMARDs

_____ Reduce immune response, increasing risk for infections

_____ Heart failure

14. Antigout drugs

_____ Reduce the amount of enzymes that convert purines in protein into uric acid

_____ To prevent gout, these drugs must be taken daily.

_____ Lower uric acid levels that occur during rapid cell destruction

Adverse Reactions to Antigout Drugs

_____ Increased risk of infection

_____ Gallstones

_____ Liver failure

PATIENT & FAMILY TEACHING

Provide a short answer to each of the following questions.

Teaching Patients and Families about NSAIDs

15. Why should NSAIDs be taken with a full glass of water?

_____

16. Contact your healthcare provider if you experience any of the following symptoms:

_____

17. How many glasses of water a day should you drink?

_____

Teaching Patients and Families about Corticosteroids

18. Why could heavy smoking be a problem?

_____

19. What are at least three symptoms that could indicate a life-threatening problem with the patient's adrenal glands?

_____

20. Why should the patient eat a diet rich in potassium and low in sodium?

_____

21. What are at least three symptoms of hypokalemia (decreased potassium in the blood)?

_____

Teaching Patients and Families about Disease-modifying Antirheumatic Drugs (DMARDs)

22. What are at least three symptoms indicating the patient may be having problems with the liver?

_____

23. What are at least three symptoms indicating the patient may have an infection?

_____

24. What should patients avoid until contacting their healthcare providers while taking DMARDs?

_____

Teaching Patients and Families about Antigout Drugs

25. How should the patient take allopurinol?

_____

26. How much liquid should the patient drink?

_____

27. What types of foods should the patient avoid?

_____

28. Which antigout drug is not impacted by meals or antacids?

_____

PRACTICE QUIZ

1. What are the five major symptoms of inflammation?
   a. Nausea, fever, warmth, swelling, loss of function
   b. Pain, redness, warmth, swelling, loss of function
   c. Nausea, redness, warmth, swelling, loss of function
   d. Pain, redness, warmth, swelling, loss of muscle control

2. How do inflammation responses within the body help injured tissue regain function?
   a. Trigger swelling around damaged joints to protect underlying tissue
   b. Prevent autoimmune diseases from developing
   c. Stimulate healthy cell growth to replace dead or damaged cells
   d. Block scar tissue development

3. What is one condition that can occur if inflammation does not go away when no longer needed or occurs when there is no injury?
   a. Serious and painful tissue damage
   b. Life-threatening infections
   c. Loss of muscle control in the affected area
   d. Inflammatory response spread to other areas within the body

4. Why is it important to monitor patients who are taking anti-inflammatory drugs?
   a. It is only necessary to monitor patients who are taking anti-inflammatory drugs on a long-term basis.
   b. Taking anti-inflammatory drugs incorrectly can lead to permanent damage to the heart and liver.
   c. Development of scar tissue while taking drugs can prevent tissue from healing.
   d. There are adverse reactions to all anti-inflammatory drugs.

5. Why do COX-1 inhibitors, such as aspirin, cause more side effects than COX-2 inhibitors?
   a. COX-1 inhibitors block the cellular COX-1, which is protective, as well as inflammation associated with COX-2.
   b. COX-1 inhibitors block white blood cells necessary for healing the inflammation.
   c. COX-1 inhibitors, unlike COX-2 inhibitors, increase bleeding risks for patients taking anticoagulants.
   d. COX-1 inhibitors frequently lead to overdoses due to their availability as over-the-counter drugs.

Chapter **12** Anti-inflammatory, Anti-arthritis, and Antigout Drugs

6. When taking the history of a patient who has just suffered an injury leading to inflammation, what question should you be certain to include to ensure your patient's safety?
   a. Ask whether the patient can safely walk on his or her own or if he or she needs assistance.
   b. Ask the patient if he or she is taking any over-the-counter drugs, including aspirin, on a regular basis.
   c. Ask the patient if he or she is prone to injuries or if this was the first time.
   d. Ask the patient if he or she is taking any pain-relief drugs obtained illegally.

7. How do corticosteroid drugs prevent or limit inflammation?
   a. Inhibit cortisol hormone secreted by the adrenal gland
   b. Increase production of white blood cells in the bone marrow
   c. Slow or stop all known pathways of inflammatory cytokine production
   d. Allow COX-1 and COX-2 enzymes to produce inflammatory mediators

8. Which of the conditions listed below are **NOT** treated by corticosteroids?
   a. Severe asthma
   b. Atrial fibrillation
   c. Systemic lupus erythematosus
   d. Acute adrenal emergencies

9. Why is it necessary for the patient to taper the dose of corticosteroids when discontinuing their use?
   a. Tapering lowers risk of infection as white blood cell production increases.
   b. Tapering allows the adrenal gland to begin producing sufficient cortisol again.
   c. Tapering prevents adverse effects such as delirium or mania.
   d. Tapering lowers the risk of developing Cushing Syndrome.

10. When assessing a patient before corticosteroid drug therapy, what is one of the most important conditions you need to identify?
    a. Ensure the patient does not have stomach issues as GI bleeding could occur.
    b. Ensure the patient is able to take the drug as prescribed as missed dosages and discontinuing the drug can have severe consequences.
    c. Ensure the patient does not have any infections as corticosteroids can reduce immunity.
    d. Ensure the patient is accurate regarding all prescribed and over-the-counter drugs he or she is currently taking.

11. How do DMARDs reduce the progression of tissue destruction in inflammatory diseases?
    a. Prevent production of cortisol
    b. Inhibit tumor necrosis factor (TNF)
    c. Increase blood flow in damaged areas
    d. Reduce pain significantly, allowing for physical therapy

12. Why do patients taking DMARDs have a risk for developing anemia and an increased risk for bleeding?
    a. Thinning of skin increases the chances of bleeding and blood loss and consequently anemia.
    b. Frequent inactivity and nausea lead to weakness and lack of nutrients entering the body.
    c. Minerals are used in tissue repair and, therefore, not available to protect the patient from other conditions such as anemia.
    d. DMARDs reduce bone marrow production of red blood cells and platelets.

13. What must patients be tested for before starting a DMARD?
    a. Hepatitis C
    b. HIV
    c. Tuberculosis
    d. Emphysema

14. What lifestyle changes can 10% of persons diagnosed with gout make to control the disease?
    a. Eat little or no shellfish, specific other fish, red and organ meats, pork, beer, and wine.
    b. Get 1 hour of moderate exercise on a daily basis.
    c. Remove all dairy, wheat, and sugar from the diet.
    d. Do weight training three times per week.

15. Which of the following statements describe how gout affects the body?
    a. Reaction to proteins within the blood, creating joint inflammation
    b. Inability of kidney to efficiently eliminate urine, causing excess fluid and swelling in joints
    c. Increase of uric acid crystals that are deposited into the joints
    d. Swelling in joints due to leaking of fluid from capillaries

13 Drugs for Gastroinstestinal Issues

KEY TERMS

Match the term with the correct definition.

Definitions

1. _____ A category of drugs used to help neutralize gastric acid and reduce symptoms of indigestion and heartburn

2. _____ A category of drugs used to prevent and treat nausea and vomiting

3. _____ Drugs that reduce or stop loose, watery stools and help to restore normal bowel movements

4. _____ Drugs that are either natural or synthetic forms of THC that reduce nausea and vomiting by binding to both cannabinoid receptors in the chemoreceptor trigger zone (CTZ) and by preventing serotonin 5-HT$_3$ from binding to its receptors in the CTZ

5. _____ A class of drugs that protect the lining of the stomach and prevent further damage

6. _____ A class of drugs that inhibit the binding of histamine to H$_2$-receptors on the parietal cells in the stomach, thereby decreasing gastric acid secretions

7. _____ A class of drugs that promote bowel movements by stimulating peristalsis, increasing the bulk of the stool, or by softening the stool

8. _____ A class of antidiarrheal drugs that reduce GI motility and increase the ability of the intestine to absorb water

9. _____ A type of antiemetic drug that reduces nausea and vomiting by blocking dopamine receptors in the CTZ

10. _____ A class of drugs that increase contraction of the upper GI tract, including the stomach and the small intestines, to move contents more quickly through the tract by blocking dopamine (D2) receptors in the CTZ and the intestinal track

11. _____ A class of drugs that bind to the proton pump of the parietal cells in the stomach, which blocks acid secretion into the stomach

12. _____ A class of antiemetic drugs that reduce or halt nausea and vomiting by blocking 5-HT$_3$ receptors in the intestinal tract and the CTZ so serotonin cannot activate these receptors

13. _____ A class of antiemetic drugs that block the substance P/neurokinin$_1$ (NK$_1$) receptors in the CTZ, preventing the substance P and neurokinin that are released from cells exposed to chemotherapy and damage in surgery from binding to and triggering the CTZ

Terms

A. Substance P/neurokinin$_1$ (NK$_1$) receptor antagonists
B. Serotonin (5-HT$_3$) receptor antagonists
C. Proton pump inhibitors
D. Promotility drugs
E. Antiemetic
F. Antidiarrheal
G. Antacids
H. Phenothiazines
I. Opioid agonists
J. Laxatives
K. Histamine H$_2$-receptor antagonists
L. Cytoprotective drugs
M. Cannabinoids

DEFINITIONS

Antiemetic and Promotility Drugs

14. Complete the table.

NAMES	ACTIONS	SIDE EFFECTS	ADVERSE EFFECTS
Serotonin (5-HT$_3$) receptor antagonists	Antiemetic drugs that reduce or halt nausea and vomiting by blocking 5-HT$_3$ receptors in the intestinal tract and the CTZ so serotonin cannot activate these receptors	_____ _____ _____ _____ _____ _____ _____ _____	_____ _____ _____ _____ _____
Substance P/neurokinin$_1$ (NK$_1$) receptor antagonists	_____ _____ _____ _____ _____	Fatigue, diarrhea, headache and dizziness. The patient may experience mild hiccoughs, flatulence, and sweating.	_____ _____ _____ _____
_____	Antiemetic drug that reduces nausea and vomiting by blocking dopamine (D$_2$) receptors in the CTZ of the brain. Approved to reduce nausea and vomiting from many problems except morning sickness associated with pregnancy	_____ _____ _____ _____ _____ _____ _____ _____ _____	Tardive dyskinesia, acute dystonia, and even neuroleptic malignant syndrome. Blood abnormalities are possible. Patients with cardiovascular disease can experience angina, tachycardia, and/or orthostatic hypotension.

60

NAMES	ACTIONS	SIDE EFFECTS	ADVERSE EFFECTS
Cannabinoids	Drugs that are either natural or synthetic forms of THC that reduce nausea and vomiting by binding to both cannabinoid receptors in the CTZ and by preventing serotonin (5-HT$_3$) from binding to its receptors in the CTZ	_____ _____ _____ _____ _____ _____ _____ _____ _____	_____ _____ _____ _____ _____ _____ _____ _____ _____
Promotility drugs	_____ _____ _____ _____ _____ _____ _____ _____ _____ _____ _____ _____ _____	_____ _____ _____ _____ _____ _____ _____ _____ _____ _____	Can cause depression and even suicidal ideation, seizures, blood disorders, cardiac dysrhythmias and heart failure. Symptoms similar to Parkinson disease, including tremor, bradykinesia, and mask-like faces. Severe adverse effects include tardive dyskinesia, akathesia, and acute dystonia.

TEACHING PATIENTS AND FAMILIES ABOUT ANTIEMETIC AND PROMOTILITY DRUGS

Fill in the blank for each of the topics below that describe the type of information patients and their families need to be aware of when taking antiemetic and promotility drugs.

15. Tell the pharmacist or your healthcare provider about any other _____ or prescribed drugs you are

taking in order to avoid _____.

16. Avoid driving, operating any machinery, or _____ while taking antiemetic drugs because they may impair your judgment and reflexes.

17. It is best to take the antiemetic drug for nausea rather than waiting until after you have had an _____

_____.

18. Do not use any alcohol or drugs with _____ while taking antiemetics.

19. If you are taking the oral solution of _____, avoid shaking the mixture. You can gently swirl the mixture and turn over the measuring cup or syringe.

Chapter **13 Drugs for Gastroinstestinal Issues**

20. Tell patients to _____ if they experience dizziness when taking phenothiazines.

21. Phenothiazines can decrease your ability to _____, and patients may become more sensitive to the sun.

    Advise patients to avoid _____ and _____.

22. Patients taking phenothiazines should contact their healthcare provider immediately if they experience any muscle

    spasms (particularly of the neck muscles); involuntary movements of the _____, _____, _____; or any unusual restlessness.

23. Patients should be taught to contact their healthcare provider immediately if they experience _____

    or _____ when taking promotility drugs.

24. An increase of _____, _____ or _____ could be a sign of a more serious illness when taking promotility drugs, and patients should report these to their healthcare provider.

25. Some men may experience _____ or _____; some women may experience

    _____. These are generally reversible within a few weeks to a few months.

DRUGS FOR PEPTIC ULCER DISEASE AND GASTROESOPHAGEAL REFLUX DISEASE

Match the drug to the correct action, side effect, or adverse effect. Some answers will be used more than once.

Correct Actions, Side Effects, and Adverse Effects

Drugs

A. Antacids
B. Histamine H_2-receptor antagonists
C. Proton pump inhibitors (PPIs)
D. Cytoprotective drugs

26. _____ Protects the lining of the stomach and protects it from further damage

27. _____ Magnesium-based versions of this drug are usually related to hypermagnesemia, low blood pressure, and low heart rate. Calcium-containing versions can cause bone pain, kidney stones, and in severe cases, cardiac dysrhythmias. Aluminum-containing versions can cause mood changes, confusion, osteoporosis, and hypercalcemia.

28. _____ Binds to the H_2 receptor in the stomach cells, leading to a decrease in production of basal and nighttime gastric acid. It also decreases the amount of gastric acid released with meals and with substances such as caffeine.

29. _____ Side effects include headache, mild abdominal pain, nausea and vomiting, flatulence, diarrhea or constipation, and increased sensitivity to light. Less common side effects include dizziness, anxiety, or mild rash.

30. _____ Drugs that neutralize hydrochloric acid (HCl) increase gastric pH, which in turn reduces gastric irritation. Only provide temporary relief.

31. _____ Adverse reactions are rare and include severe allergic reactions, a variety of blood disorders, and cardiac dysrhythmias. While the reason is not fully known, patients may also be at risk for pneumonia.

32. _____ Help heal gastric ulcers and reduce symptoms of gastroesophageal reflux disease (GERD) by stopping the acid secretory pump that is located within the gastric parietal cell membrane, therefore reducing the amount of acid secreted into the stomach

33. _____ Headache, nausea, diarrhea or constipation, and mild abdominal pain. Some patients may have mental status changes including confusion, anxiety, or depression.

34. _____ Brands with magnesium can cause diarrhea; brands with calcium or aluminum can cause constipation. Other side effects include loss of appetite, frequent burping, nausea and vomiting, fatigue, and weight loss.

35. _____ Severe allergic reactions, pancreatitis, and blood abnormalities including thrombocytopenia and hemolytic anemia. May have increased risk for osteoporosis and bone fracture with long-term use.

TEACHING PATIENTS AND FAMILIES ABOUT DRUGS FOR PEPTIC ULCER DISEASE AND GASTROESOPHEGAL REFLUX

Match the class of drugs to the information that is important to teach patients and families. Some descriptions may have more than one answer.

Patient Information

36. _____ Wear sunscreen and protective clothing because your skin may be more sensitive to light.

37. _____ These drugs do not cure ulcers, but they do reduce acid in your stomach so that the ulcer can heal.

38. _____ These drugs are for temporary relief. If symptoms persist after 2 weeks or after completing a prescribed amount, contact your healthcare provider.

39. _____ Take the drug 1 hour after meals and before bedtime.

40. _____ Ask your family members to observe you for any changes in mental status such as confusion or anxiety and depression.

41. _____ Once-a-day dosing of this drug is best taken at bedtime to reduce symptoms of acid reflux at night.

42. _____ These drugs neutralize gastric acids and are typically most beneficial if given between meals and at bedtime.

43. _____ Do not drive or operate heavy machinery until you see how the drug affects you.

44. _____ Diarrhea and constipation are common side effects. Contact your healthcare provider if severe.

45. _____ If this drug is in chewable form, chew completely and follow with a glass of water. If liquid, be sure and shake well.

46. _____ Avoid driving or using heavy machinery while using this drug as it may cause dizziness.

47. _____ Avoid cigarette smoking because it increases gastric acid production and can decrease the effectiveness of this drug.

48. _____ If you are taking other drugs, it is usually best to take them 1 hour before or 2 hours after taking this drug.

Class of Drugs

A. Antacids
H. Histamine H_2-receptor antagonists
P. Proton pump inhibitors (PPIs)

DRUGS FOR CONSTIPATION AND DIARRHEA

Laxatives

Fill in the blanks for each topic below to describe the uses, side effects, and adverse effects for patients using laxatives.

49. Laxatives are a class of drugs that promote bowel movements by stimulating _____, increasing the _____ of the _____, or by _____ the _____.

50. Laxatives are generally for _____ but are also used for cleansing the bowel before a(n) _____, _____, or _____ procedure.

51. Describe how each type of laxative works to help relieve constipation.
    a. Bulk-forming laxatives

    _____

    _____

    _____

    _____

    b. Lubricant laxatives

    _____

    _____

    _____

    _____

    c. Stool softeners

    _____

    _____

    _____

    _____

    d. Osmotic laxative

    _____

    _____

    _____

    e. Stimulant or irritant laxatives may be used when rapid relief is desired.

    _____

    _____

    _____

    _____

52. The most common side effects of laxatives are GI symptoms such as _____,

    _____, _____, and _____.

Match the laxatives with the adverse reactions:

Adverse Reactions	Laxatives
53. _____ Rarely, a condition called *lipid pneumonia* can occur by inhalation of fat-containing substances such as mineral oil.	A. Bulk-forming laxatives
54. _____ Can produce fluid and electrolyte disturbance if used daily or in patients with renal or cardiac impairment	B. Stool softeners
55. _____ May produce decreased absorption of nutrients and fat-soluble vitamins	C. Lubricants
56. _____ Inhaling the psyllium dust particles can cause hypersensitivity reactions	D. Osmotic laxatives
57. _____ Patients who do not take the drug with enough water (at least 8–12 ounces of fluid) are at risk for esophageal obstruction. Swelling of the throat or choking might occur.	E. Stimulant laxatives
58. _____ Severe allergic reactions are possible.	
59. _____ May produce muscle weakness (following excessive use of laxatives), dermatitis, pruritus, alkalosis, and electrolyte imbalance (with excessive use)	

TEACHING PATIENTS AND FAMILIES ABOUT LAXATIVES

Fill in the blanks for the topics below to describe information important to teach patients and families about laxative use.

60. Most laxatives are recommended for _____ use only. Contact your healthcare provider if you require laxatives on a regular basis or do not have relief with the over-the-counter drugs.

61. Some laxatives are high in _____ or in _____. Make sure to read the labels carefully if you are on a special diet.

62. Laxatives are not a substitute for good bowel habits including _____ activity and a diet that

    includes high-fiber foods such as _____, _____, and _____.

63. Many types of drugs increase the risk of _____. If you are taking a drug that causes _____, contact your healthcare provider to determine the best type of laxative for you.

64. Never take a laxative to treat _____ _____ _____ because the drug may make conditions worse.

65. The onset of action of laxatives varies according to the specific drug category. These drugs can work in as short a

    period of time as _____or as long as _____. Knowing the expected onset will help you plan.

ANTIDIARRHEALS

Fill in the blanks for each topic below to describe the uses, side effects, and adverse effects of antidiarrheals.

66. Antidiarrheals are drugs that reduce or stop _____, _____ _____ and help to restore normal bowel movements.

67. Three general drug classes are used to treat these problems: _____, _____

    or _____.

68. Anticholinergics reduce GI tract _____ and intestinal _____, _____ production, and

    _____ motility and thus reduce the associated pain.

69. The antispasmodic drugs reduce _____ in the GI tract. This causes decreased cramping, bloating, and diarrhea.

70. Opioid agonists are effective for diarrhea but do not have the _____or other opioid-like effects. They do however, reduce GI motility and increase the ability of the intestine to absorb water. Stools then increase bulk, and the patient loses fewer fluids and _____.

71. A fourth drug for diarrhea is _____. While the action is not fully understood, this drug may prevent the attachment of certain organisms to the _____ and provide a protective coating. It is used to treat _____ diarrhea and diarrhea caused by _____. It is also used to prevent _____ diarrhea.

72. The most common side effects of antidiarrheals include _____, _____, _____ and _____. Other possible side effects may be dizziness or drowsiness.

73. _____ have many drug interactions that can cause adverse reactions. _____ taken with other opioid drugs can increase the opioid effect.

74. List at least three important topics that are important information to teach patients and families about antidiarrheals.

1. _____

_____

2. _____

_____

3. _____

_____

PRACTICE QUIZ

1. What issues are patients at most risk for when experiencing nausea and vomiting?
   a. Dizziness, drowsiness, and mental confusion
   b. Dehydration, weight loss, and electrolyte imbalance
   c. Swelling of the throat, choking, and dehydration
   d. Diarrhea, weight loss, and electrolyte imbalance

2. All the serotonin (5-HT$_3$) receptor antagonists have what ending in their generic names?
   a. "tidine"
   b. "noid"
   c. "setron"
   d. "prazole"

3. Why are drugs that decrease prostaglandins such as corticosteroids and NSAIDs harmful to the stomach?
   a. Decreased prostaglandins cause diarrhea, nausea, and vomiting.
   b. Prostaglandins are necessary for proper digestion.
   c. A decrease in prostaglandins will eventually cause bone loss and osteoporosis.
   d. Prostaglandins maintain good blood flow to the stomach, keeping tissues oxygenated.

4. All the histamine H$_2$ receptor antagonists have what ending in their generic names?
   a. "tidine"
   b. "noid"
   c. "setron"
   d. "prazole"

5. What issues are older adults more likely to experience as side effects of H$_2$ blockers compared with younger adults?
   a. Gastric ulcers
   b. Confusion and dizziness
   c. Nausea and vomiting
   d. Constipation

6. All the proton pump inhibitors have what ending in their generic names?
   a. "tidine"
   b. "noid"
   c. "setron"
   d. "prazole"

7. Why would a healthcare provider **NOT** provide an antidiarrheal to treat a patient's diarrhea?
   a. When patient does not have irritable bowel syndrome
   b. To help patient rid the body of an infection if the infection is causing the diarrhea
   c. To avoid side effects of antidiarrheals
   d. When patient is not experiencing dehydration

8. Which of the following is not an example of direct stimuli that can send messages to the vomiting center to cause nausea and vomiting?
   a. Cerebral cortex
   b. Vestibular apparatus
   c. Sensory organs
   d. Chemoreceptor trigger zone (CTZ)

9. Which class of antiemetic drugs is also called dopamine antagonists?
   a. Cannabinoids
   b. Substance P antagonists
   c. Serotonin (5-HT$_3$) receptor antagonists
   d. Phenothiazines

10. Antidepressants and St. John's Wort should not be taken with which drugs?
    a. Cannabinoids
    b. Substance P antagonists
    c. Serotonin (5-HT$_3$) receptor antagonists
    d. Phenothiazines

11. When gastric distress causes destruction to the protective mucosal lining of the stomach, what can be produced if the lining is not repaired or gastric acid reduced?
    a. Duodenal and gastric ulcers
    b. Nausea and vomiting
    c. Constipation
    d. Diarrhea

12. What bacteria may also cause peptic ulcers?
    a. *Clostridium difficile*
    b. *E. coli*
    c. *H. pylori*
    d. *Salmonella*

13. Which symptom is **NOT** a symptom of constipation?
    a. Less than three bowel movements per week
    b. Harder stools than normal
    c. Bowels still feeling full after a bowel movement
    d. Electrolyte imbalance

14. What is the best treatment for constipation?
    a. Cytoprotective drugs
    b. Healthy diet, adequate hydration, physical exercise
    c. Stool-softening drugs
    d. Osmotic drugs

15. When a patient has diarrhea due to a bacterial infection and cannot take antidiarrheals because it would slow down the body's ability to get rid of the organism, what is your role in supporting the patient?
    a. Diet and nutrition counseling
    b. Assisting in toileting
    c. Making sure that patient has adequate hydration and skin care to prevent irritation to anus
    d. Providing drugs to relieve pain and anxiety

Drugs Affecting the Hematologic System

MATCHING

Match the drugs listed in the left column with the drug categories on the right.

Drugs

1. _____ Reteplase

2. _____ Heparin

3. _____ Darbepoietin alpha

4. _____ Apixaban

5. _____ Aspirin

6. _____ Enoxaparin

7. _____ Clopidogrel

8. _____ Alteplase

9. _____ Rivaroxaban

10. _____ Warfarin

Drug Categories

A. Platelet inhibitors
B. Direct thrombin inhibitors
C. Indirect thrombin inhibitors
D. Vitamin K antagonist
E. Fibrinolytics
F. Erythropoiesis-stimulating agents

CATEGORIES	SIDE EFFECTS	ADVERSE EFFECTS
Fibrinolytic drugs	Bleeding Bleeding of the gums, or injection, or IV sites Low blood pressure (hypotension)	_____ _____ _____ _____ _____ _____ _____ _____
_____	Pain at the injection sites Generalized body aches and pain Skin rash Redness or warmth at the injection site	Higher risk for hypertension, blood clots, stroke, and myocardial infarction (heart attack) Increased tumor growth in some cancers Severe allergic reactions

MULTIPLE CHOICE

For each of the drug categories listed below, check all items that describe what should be taught to patients and families.

28. Platelet inhibitors

    _____ Take these drugs at least 2 hours before meals.

    _____ Look for symptoms of bleeding.

    _____ Avoid foods, supplements, and over-the-counter (OTC) drugs that can interfere with drugs.

    _____ Do not stop taking these drugs for any reason.

29. Direct thrombin inhibitors

    _____ Look for signs of abnormal bleeding, including heavy menses.

    _____ Look for allergic reactions that include shortness of breath, facial swelling, rash, or hives.

    _____ Teach patients to take aspirin for aches and pains rather than other OTC drugs.

    _____ Pills should be removed from packaging and placed in plastic pill containers.

30. Indirect thrombin inhibitors

    _____ Look for signs of abnormal bleeding, including heavy menses.

    _____ Look for allergic reactions that include shortness of breath, facial swelling, rash, or hives.

    _____ Avoid aspirin or NSAIDs because of increased excessive bleeding risks.

    _____ Patient with latex allergies must find an alternative to these drugs.

31. Vitamin K antagonist

    _____ Patients **MUST** ensure they eat a sufficient amount of green, leafy vegetables to replace Vitamin K deficiency.

    _____ Teach patients to keep all appointments for international normalized ratio (INR) laboratory tests, which determine proper dosage.

    _____ To avoid excessive bleeding, patient should not take aspirin or NSAIDs.

32. Fibrinolytics

    _____ Teach patient and family to give this drug at home.

    _____ Ensure patient and family understand purpose, risks, and benefits.

    _____ Inform the patient and family what symptoms to report after this drug has been given.

33. Erythropoeisis-stimulating agents (ESAs)

_____ The patient should weigh daily and report gains of 2 pounds within 24 hours or 4 pounds in a week due to possible water retention.

_____ Ensure patient that chest pains are normal side effects when taking this drug and there is no need to report this to the healthcare provider.

_____ Patient must inform healthcare provider if pregnant, breast-feeding, or planning to become pregnant.

PRACTICE QUIZ

1. Why is it important for blood to flow freely through blood vessels?
   a. Distributes waste products in the blood stream to organs such as kidneys
   b. Provides cells with oxygen and nutrients
   c. Protects cells from excesses of enzymes
   d. Prevents clotting of blood

2. What is the most common reason for blood beginning to clot?
   a. Due to deficiency of the thrombin enzyme
   b. Excessive Vitamin K within the blood stream
   c. Damage to the blood vessels or tissues
   d. Lack of sufficient red blood cells

3. If the arteries become plugged with thrombi (clots of fibrin, platelets, and cholesterol), what can happen to the body's tissues?
   a. Oxygen is prohibited from reaching the tissues, which may result in death.
   b. Emboli can break off and cause bleeding in other parts of the body.
   c. Clots can damage legs or ankles and cause permanent neuropathy.
   d. Glucose is prohibited from reaching the muscles, which may cause weakness.

4. How do anticoagulants interfere in the clotting process?
   a. Thin the blood
   b. Reduce or prevent new clots from forming
   c. Dissolve existing clots
   d. Prevent clots from breaking off as emboli

5. How do fibrinolytic drugs interfere in the clotting process?
   a. Prevent plasminogen from converting to plasmin
   b. Provide plasma proteins to protect the tissue
   c. Emergency drug carried by patients to use when they determine clot is forming
   d. Dissolve and break down existing blood clots

6. How does platelet aggregation protect the body when it is injured?
   a. Platelet aggregation prevents clots in the cardiovascular system.
   b. Platelet aggregation keeps the blood thin so clots are unable to be formed when there are injuries.
   c. Platelets aggregate and seal the entry to the vascular system to prevent blood from accessing the body tissues.
   d. Platelets aggregate and inhibit clots from breaking off and moving to other parts of the body.

7. What is a common sign of excessive bleeding that patients need to notice?
   a. Frequent heavy nosebleeds
   b. Bleeding from the gums when brushing teeth
   c. Bleeding around the cuticles when washing hands or feet
   d. Unusually reddened eyes

8. Which of the following can increase bleeding or decrease the effectiveness of an anticoagulant drug?
   a. Red meat
   b. Diet cola
   c. St. John's Wort
   d. Acetaminophen

9. Which of the following drug types is frequently given for atrial fibrillation?
   a. Direct thrombin inhibitors
   b. Indirect thrombin inhibitors
   c. Vitamin K antagonist
   d. Fibrinolytics

10. What is low-molecular heparin especially used to prevent?
    a. Venous thromboembolism
    b. Pulmonary embolism
    c. Cardiac arrest
    d. Dysrhythmia

11. What is the most commonly used blood test for determining the therapeutic range for heparin?
    a. Activated partial thromboplastin time
    b. Prothrombin time
    c. International normalized ratio
    d. PT/INR

12. Within how many hours after the onset of a stroke must fibrinolytics be started to dissolve the blood clot blocking the artery?
    a. Within 12 hours
    b. Within 3 hours
    c. Within 6 hours
    d. Within 4-8 hours

13. What happens when red blood cell (RBC) counts fall due to anemia?
    a. The liver secretes the hormone thrombopoietin, which travels to the bone marrow.
    b. Patients must be treated with supplements to increase RBC production and receive further treatment with ESAs.
    c. The kidneys secrete the hormone erythropoietin, which stimulates production of RBCs.
    d. Patients require a bone-marrow transplant and injections of ESAs.

14. Which of the following drug types can help reduce the need for transfusions?
    a. Indirect thrombin inhibitors
    b. Vitamin K antagonist
    c. Fibrinolytics
    d. Erythropoiesis-stimulating agents

15. What should patients taking anticoagulants do before dental surgical procedures?
    a. Discontinue the drug before surgery to avoid bleeding issues.
    b. Ensure all procedures are done within a fully equipped surgical facility.
    c. Discontinue the drug after the surgery for at least 72 hours.
    d. Work with healthcare provider to obtain another drug less likely to cause bleeding issues.

73

15 Drugs for Immunization and Immunomodulation

TYPES OF IMMUNITY

Indicate for each description in the left column what type of immunity is applicable.

Descriptions

1. _____ A 30-year-old man is bitten by a rabid raccoon. He had not been previously vaccinated for rabies. He receives a series of injections that contain antibodies created by other individuals who had rabies. Once the shots are discontinued, his body destroys the antibodies that were not created in his body.

2. _____ A woman and her infant are exposed to a disease for which the woman has developed antibodies within her body. She is currently breast-feeding the infant, and the infant resists the disease as well.

3. _____ A patient who previously had strep throat is exposed again. Her body already has antibodies prepared to destroy the bacteria, and the effects of the disease are much less severe. She develops more antibodies, and when she is exposed again, the bacteria are destroyed before causing any disease.

4. _____ A 60-year-old man receives a pneumonia vaccine, which contains a few microorganisms of the disease, and his body creates protective antibodies to the pneumococcal bacteria without actually having been exposed to the disease. He will likely need booster shots to ensure his antibodies remain active.

5. _____ A patient is exposed to the *Streptococcus pyogenes* bacteria (strep throat), and immediately her body begins developing antibodies to fight off the cells that do not contain her genetic code.

Types of Immunity

A. Innate immunity
B. Natural acquired active immunity
C. Natural acquired passive immunity
D. Artificial acquired active immunity
E. Artificial acquired passive immunity

NURSING RESPONSIBILITY FOR GIVING VACCINATIONS

6. Number each of the items listed below in the order you would perform the action.

_____ Unpack and store vials in designated area with refrigerator separate from other drugs.

_____ Observe the patient for any immediate reactions.

_____ Inject the vaccine using recommended technique and site.

_____ Check the expiration date on the vaccine vial.

_____ Draw up appropriate dose.

_____ Document all required information.

_____ Tell patient what side effects could be expected.

_____ Ask the patient if he ever had a reaction to the vaccine or components.

VACCINATION SCHEDULES

7. For each age shown on the timeline, write above or below the timeline the letter associated with the recommended vaccination(s) and/or booster(s).
   a. DTaP
   b. DTaP booster
   c. Tdap
   d. Tdap booster
   e. Pneumonia
   f. Influenza
   g. Shingles

| 2 mos | 4 mos | 6 mos | 15–18 mos | 4–6 yrs | 11–12 yrs | 19 yrs | 19, 29, 39 etc. | 65 yrs |

8. For each of the diseases listed below, indicate whether a vaccine should be given in (a) childhood, (b) adulthood, or (c) based on vocation/travel.

   _____ Malaria

   _____ HPV

   _____ Typhoid

   _____ Hepatitis A and B

   _____ Measles, mumps, rubella

   _____ Polio

   _____ Pertussis

   _____ Rabies

9. Select which of the following vaccines can be given to women **DURING** pregnancy.

   _____ Measles, mumps, rubella (MMR)

   _____ Seasonal influenza

   _____ Tdap

   _____ Chicken pox

   _____ Polio

IDENTIFYING SELECTIVE IMMUNOSUPPRESSANT DRUGS

Match each drug listed in the left column to one of the drug categories listed in the right column.

Drugs	Drug Categories
10. _____ Mycophenolate	A. Antiproliferative drugs
11. _____ Cyclosporine	B. Calcineurin drugs
12. _____ Sirolimus	
13. _____ Azathioprine	
14. _____ Tacrolimus	
15. _____ Everolimus	

FILL IN THE BLANK

Using the list of drugs from the exercise above, fill in the name of the drug to match the descriptions.

16. _____ selectively suppresses T and B lymphocyte activity by inhibiting an enzyme needed for lymphocyte reproduction and prevents T-cell activation.

17. _____ inhibits T-cell activation and reproduction, blocking the mTOR signal pathways that promote completion of cell division for T cells. Fewer T cells lead to less tumor necrosis factor and other substances that can attack normal tissues and transplanted organs.

18. _____ inhibits the mTOR pathway so lymphocyte cell division and growth are reduced. It is more specific against immune system cells that attack normal self-cells and transplanted organs than general antiproliferative drugs.

19. _____ and _____ are calcineurin inhibitors and work by forming a complex around the normal calcineurin present inside T lymphocytes, preventing the calcineurin from activating those cells. With less ability to be activated, the T cells are not able to attack and damage transplanted tissues and organs.

TRUE OR FALSE

Indicate whether each of the following statements is True (T) or False (F).

20. _____ Selective immunosuppressants are safe for use even if a patient has a systemic infection.

21. _____ Tacrolimus can cause diabetes mellitus.

22. _____ Sirolimus is the only selective immunosuppressant that increases blood cholesterol levels.

23. _____ Calcineurin inhibitors increase blood cholesterol and blood glucose levels.

24. _____ Patients taking selective immunosuppressants are at an increased risk for cancer.

25. _____ Phlebitis and thrombosis can be adverse effects when patients are taking calcineurin inhibitors orally.

26. _____ Liver failure can occur with all selective immunosuppressants.

27. _____ Antiproliferatives are the only category of selective immunosuppressants that can cause imbalances of potassium, phosphorus, and magnesium.

28. _____ Patients taking selective immunosuppressants should ensure they are vaccinated with all vaccination options to prevent infections.

SHORT ANSWER

Answer the questions below, indicating how you would teach patients and their families about the following concerns.

29. What are at least five signs that may be indicative of a potential infection that should be monitored daily by patients or their families?

_____

_____

30. What are at least three signs that may be indicative of potential liver toxicity and should be monitored daily by patients or their families?

_____

_____

31. Name two substances the patient should avoid to prevent liver damage when taking immunosuppressant drugs?

_____

_____

32. Why is it important for the patient to take the drugs exactly as prescribed?

_____

_____

33. Describe how to direct the patient to effectively give the oral suspensions of sirolimus or cyclosporine.

_____

_____

_____

_____

34. If taking sirolimus as well as cyclosporine, when should drugs be given to ensure the best effect?

_____

_____

35. Why should sirolimus or tacrolimus not be taken with grapefruit juice?

_____

_____

PRACTICE QUIZ

1. Which of the following best describes innate immunity?
   a. Occurs when all vaccinations have been taken as scheduled as children, and the individual is protected by antibodies
   b. Occurs when the body recognizes foreign cells invading the body and takes action by developing antibodies
   c. Occurs when the body is invaded by common diseases, and family members or close acquaintances are not infected
   d. Occurs when adult vaccinations are taken on a regular basis

2. Which of the following best describes acquired immunity?
   a. Occurs when the body is exposed to microorganisms after already having built antigens to destroy it
   b. Occurs from vaccinations
   c. Occurs when newborns acquire it from the mother in vitro
   d. Occurs when a current infection within the body prevents other infections from taking hold

3. Immunity acquired through vaccinations is referred to as which of the following types of immunity?
   a. Natural acquired active immunity
   b. Natural acquired passive immunity
   c. Artificial acquired active immunity
   d. Artificial acquired passive immunity

4. Why do vaccinations target B cells to stimulate antibody production?
   a. B cells are located in the lymphatic system.
   b. B cells are capable of helping the body develop natural immunity.
   c. B cells are the most prolific cells found in the body.
   d. B cells are the only white blood cells (WBC) that can form antibodies in response to the vaccine.

5. What is the difference between vaccination and immunization?
   a. Vaccinations refer to shots with live cultures; immunizations refer to shots containing antibodies.
   b. Vaccinations are generally for children, and immunizations refer to adults.
   c. Vaccinations are the actual shots, and immunization is what occurs within the body.
   d. Vaccinations and immunizations are used interchangeably.

6. What types of vaccines are composed of chemically modified microorganisms?
   a. Inactivated vaccines
   b. Attenuated vaccines
   c. Toxoid vaccines
   d. Biosynthetic vaccines

7. What types of vaccines are composed of microorganisms that have been killed?
   a. Inactivated vaccines
   b. Attenuated vaccines
   c. Toxoid vaccines
   d. Biosynthetic vaccines

8. What types of vaccines are composed of genetically engineered microorganisms?
   a. Inactivated vaccines
   b. Attenuated vaccines
   c. Toxoid vaccines
   d. Biosynthetic vaccines

9. What types of vaccines are composed of weakened but live organisms?
   a. Inactivated vaccines
   b. Attenuated vaccines
   c. Toxoid vaccines
   d. Biosynthetic vaccines

10. What occurs in the body when an individual develops an autoimmune disorder?
   a. The body keeps developing antibodies after the foreign microorganism has been destroyed, and the antibodies enter the bloodstream.
   b. Autoimmune disorders occur after receiving a blood transfusion, and foreign substances attack the organs.
   c. The immune system views normal body tissue as foreign and attacks it.
   d. The immune system has been suppressed due to chemical substances and prevents appropriate response when a foreign substance invades the body.

11. Why are selective immunosuppressant drugs preferred to nonselective immunosuppressant drugs for patients with autoimmune diseases?
   a. Selective immunosuppressant drugs target the affected area, reducing infection risk.
   b. Nonselective immunosuppressant drugs are not effective for most autoimmune diseases.
   c. Selective immunosuppressant drugs are created from the patient's antibodies, which helps reduce risks of immune dysfunction.
   d. Nonselective immunosuppressant drugs must be given at significantly higher dosages.

12. In addition to autoimmune diseases such as rheumatoid arthritis, what other condition requires immunosuppressant drugs?
   a. Osteoarthritis
   b. Joint replacement
   c. Organ transplant
   d. Influenza

13. Which type of drug, when given intravenously, can cause phlebitis and/or thrombosis?
   a. Calcineurin inhibitors
   b. Antiproliferatives
   c. Toxoids
   d. Tdap

14. How do antirejection drugs work to protect a patient who has received an organ transplant?
   a. Create antibodies that ensure diseases do not impact the transplanted organ
   b. Modify toxoids chemically so they are no longer toxic
   c. Suppress the cells and factors of the immune system
   d. Prevent rejection by generating microorganisms that protect the transplanted organ

15. What is the purpose in performing an antibody titer on a patient?
   a. Detects and measures the amount of a specific antibody in the person's blood to determine the person's immunity
   b. Identifies the types of antibodies already present in a person's blood to determine which vaccines are actually needed
   c. Tests a patient with autoimmune disease to determine whether a vaccine will cause an adverse reaction
   d. Determines whether an organism that can damage tissue is in the person's system

16 Hormones and Drugs for Osteoporosis

KEY TERMS

Complete the puzzle

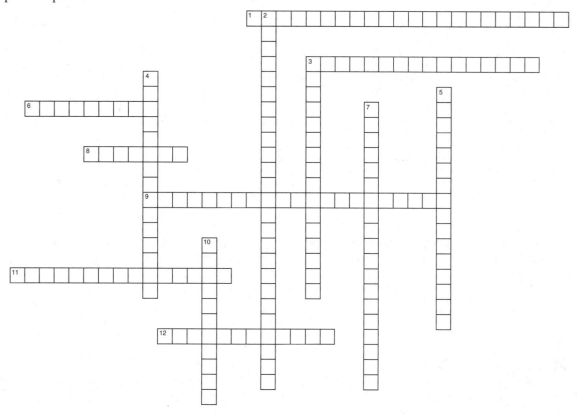

Across

1. Drugs that mimic the effect of thyroid hormones, T3 and T4, helping to regulate metabolism.
3. Thyroid-suppressing drugs that work directly in the thyroid gland to stop production of new hormones by preventing an enzyme from connecting iodine (iodide) with tyrosine to make active thyroid hormones.
6. Synthetic or natural hormones that help to develop and maintain the male sex organs at puberty and develop secondary sex characteristics in men (facial hair, deep voice, body hair, body fat distribution, and muscle development).
8. A protein secreted by an endocrine gland that changes the action of another gland or tissue, known as its target tissue.
9. The use of hormones to suppress ovulation for the intentional prevention of pregnancy.
11. Drugs similar to natural cortisol, a hormone secreted by the adrenal cortex that is essential for life.
12. The gradual loss of bone density and strength, which leads to spinal shortening and increased risk for bone fractures.

Down

2. Temporary or permanent therapy with drugs that perform the function of natural endocrine hormones.
3. Synthetic drugs with the same use and actions as androgens.
4. Calcium-modifying drugs that both prevent bones from losing calcium and increase bone density by moving blood calcium into the bone, binding to calcium in the bone, and preventing osteoclasts from destroying bone cells and reabsorbing calcium.
5. Drugs for osteoporosis that block estrogen receptors in breast and uterine tissue.
10. A hormone secreted by the adrenal cortex that regulates sodium and water balance.

79

Answer the following questions regarding endocrine glands and hormone replacement therapy (HRT).

1. Why are the endocrine glands known as "ductless" glands?

   _____

   _____

2. How do the hormones produced by the endocrine glands reach their target tissue?

   _____

   _____

3. Hormone replacement therapy (HRT) is used when endocrine glands cannot produce the adequate amount of hormone. Name the common uses of HRT.

   a. _____

   b. _____

   c. _____

   d. _____

   e. _____

4. Depending on how important the function of the hormone is to a patient's health and well-being, HRT can be used for a short time or permanently. Give an example of each circumstance.

   a. Short time _____

   b. Permanently _____

DRUGS FOR THYROID PROBLEMS

Fill in the blanks for the following statements regarding drugs for thyroid problems.

5. Name the two thyroid hormones necessary for life.

   _____

6. Name the body actions that the thyroid hormones control.

   a. _____

   b. _____

   c. _____

   d. _____

7. _____ is a condition when there is little or no production of the thyroid hormones.

8. _____ are drugs that mimic the effect of the thyroid hormones T3 and T4, helping to regulate metabolism.

9. Side effects of this class of drugs are

_____

_____

_____

_____

10. List the possible adverse reactions that may occur with thyroid hormone agonists.

    a. _____

       _____

    b. _____

       _____

11. _____ is a condition in which the thyroid gland secretes excessive amounts of thyroid hormones (T3 and T4). The most common cause is _____.

12. Severe hyperthyroidism that causes life-threatening hypertension, heart failure, and seizures is called thyroid _____ or thyroid _____. Often a _____ is the first indication of the problem. This condition is an emergency and can lead to death if the thyroid hormone levels are not decreased immediately.

13. _____ work directly in the thyroid gland to stop production of the hormones.

14. The names of these drugs are _____ and _____, which belong to the thionamide class of drugs.

15. Side effects of antithyroid drugs can include

_____

_____

_____

_____

16. List the possible adverse effects of antithyroid drugs.

    a. _____

    b. _____

    c. _____

    d. _____

Indicate which of the following statements are important to teach patients and families about thyroid hormone agonists (T) and which ones are important for antithyroid drugs (A). Some of the statements will be true for both classes of drugs.

17. _____ You must take the drug daily to maintain normal body function and not skip doses.

18. _____ Take the missed dose as soon as you remember it. However, if it is almost time for the next dose, skip the missed dose and continue your regular dosing schedule. Do not take a double dose to make up for a missed one.

19. _____ Take the drug 2 to 3 hours before a meal or taking a fiber supplement or at least 3 hours after a meal or taking the supplement because food and fiber greatly decrease absorption of the drug.

20. _____ Take only the dose that is prescribed for you, because increasing the drug too quickly can lead to adverse effects such as a heart attack or seizures.

21. _____ Keep all follow-up appointments and appointments for blood-clotting tests because these drugs increase the effectiveness of warfarin.

22. _____ If you are ill and cannot take the drug orally, contact your healthcare provider to get an injection dose of the drug.

23. _____ Go to the emergency department immediately if you start to have chest pain.

24. _____ Even if you do not notice a reduction of your symptoms in the first 1 to 2 weeks, do not increase the dosage on your own. These drugs take several weeks to be effective.

25. _____ Do not stop the drug suddenly or change the dose (up or down) without contacting your healthcare provider to prevent under dosing or overdosing.

26. _____ Check your pulse each morning before taking the drug and again each evening before going to bed. If the pulse rate becomes 20 beats higher than the normal rate for 1 week or if it becomes consistently irregular, notify your healthcare provider.

27. _____ Check the color of the roof of the mouth and the whites of your eyes daily for a yellow tinge that may indicate a liver problem. If this appears, notify your healthcare provider as soon as possible.

28. _____ Avoid situations that can lead to bleeding and other drugs that can make bleeding worse.

29. _____ Avoid crowds and people who are ill because these drugs can reduce your immunity and resistance to infection.

DRUGS FOR ADRENAL GLAND PROBLEMS

Fill in the blanks for the following statements regarding the adrenal glands.

30. What are the corticosteroid hormones produced by the cortex of the adrenal gland?

_____

31. _____ controls sodium and water balance. It is also known as a _____ because it regulates sodium.

32. _____ helps maintain critical blood glucose levels, the stress response, excitability of cardiac muscle, immunity, and blood sodium levels.

33. Cortisol was first discovered to affect blood glucose levels; it is also known as a _____.

34. _____ is a disorder in which the adrenal gland produces little or no cortisol and aldosterone.

35. When adrenal gland _____ occurs, only one hormone is oversecreted. Excessive secretion of cortisol is known as _____ or _____. Excessive secretion of aldosterone is _____.

36. _____ is the most common treatment for adrenal gland hyperfunction. Drug therapy can also be used.

Match the correct term to the descriptions regarding adrenal gland problems and the actions, side effects, and adverse reactions of the drugs used to treat those problems. You may use the terms more than once, and some descriptions may match more than one term.

Descriptions

37. _____ Conditions that cause it include autoimmune disease attacking and destroying the adrenal glands, adrenalectomy, abdominal radiation therapy, and reduced function of the anterior pituitary gland. Major problems are hypoglycemia, salt wasting, hypotension, weakness, and high blood potassium levels.

38. _____ The most common cause of this condition is an adrenal gland tumor. Sometimes a problem in the pituitary gland is responsible.

39. _____ Both of these can cause the adverse effect of adrenal insufficiency.

40. _____ Used for hormone replacement therapy, but their most common use is as a powerful anti-inflammatory drug.

41. _____ A steroid-production inhibitor that works by directly preventing adrenal gland production of cortisol and other adrenal cortex hormones.

42. _____ Drugs that act just like natural cortisol. They have some effect on sodium balance, so most patients with adrenal gland hypofunction only need hormone replacement therapy with these.

43. _____ This drug works by blocking corticosteroid receptors. Although this does not reduce cortisol levels, it does inhibit cortisol responses in different tissues.

44. _____ A synthetic drug that acts like natural aldosterone. With the use of this drug, more sodium is retained to prevent excessive sodium wasting, and more potassium is excreted to prevent dangerously high blood potassium levels. So, it helps prevent hyponatremia, hyperkalemia, and hypotension.

45. _____ Drug therapy for this condition focuses on reducing potassium levels and relies on spironolactone (Aldactone, Spironol, Novo-Spiroton), a potassium-sparing diuretic.

46. _____ Side effects include hypertension, edema formation, low blood potassium levels, and high blood sodium levels. The cause of these problems is the drug's action on fluid and electrolyte balance.

47. _____ Allergic reaction can occur. Emergency help is needed for hives; difficult breathing; and swelling of the face, lips, tongue, or throat. Used to induce abortions and can cause pregnancy loss.

48. _____ Congestive heart failure (CHF) is a serious adverse effect of this drug. It requires that the drug dose be either reduced or stopped.

49. _____ Causes nausea, vomiting, skin rashes, and dizziness. This drug can also cause bloody urine (hematuria).

50. _____ Causes nausea, vomiting, skin rashes, and dizziness. This drug can also cause menstrual irregularities.

Terms
A. Glucocorticoids, especially prednisone
B. Fludrocortisone (Florinef)
C. Mitotane (Lysodren)
D. Mifepristone (Korlym)
E. Adrenal gland hypofunction
F. Adrenal gland hyperfunction (hypercortisolism, Cushing disease, hyperaldosteronism)

TEACHING PATIENTS AND FAMILIES ABOUT DRUGS FOR ADRENAL PROBLEMS

Fill in the blanks for each of the topics below that describe important information the patient and their families should be aware of when taking drugs for adrenal problems.

51. Take _____ at the same time daily with food to prevent _____ problems.

52. Weigh yourself daily and keep a record because adrenal gland hypofunction drugs can cause fluid retention with

_____.

53. Immediately report a weight gain of ___ lb in a day or ____ lb in a week to the healthcare provider when taking adrenal gland hypofunction drugs.

54. Keep all appointments for laboratory blood work because adrenal gland hyperfunction drugs alter blood levels of

_____ and _____.

55. When taking drugs for adrenal gland hyperfunction, report symptoms of adrenal insufficiency to your healthcare provider immediately. These include

_____

_____

56. Take adrenal gland hyperfunction drugs with food because they all can cause _____, _____, and other gastrointestinal upsets.

57. If you are a sexually active woman in your childbearing years, use two reliable forms of _____

while taking _____ because this drug can cause a pregnancy loss.

DRUGS FOR SEX HORMONE REPLACEMENT AND CONTRACEPTION

Fill in the blanks for the topics below regarding the uses and actions of sex hormone replacement and contraception.

58. _____ hormone replacement therapy (HRT) during the _____ period is the replacement of naturally secreted _____ and _____ with hormones given in the form of a drug.

59. Oral contraceptives provide enough _____ to interfere with feedback and decrease the body's natural production of estrogen and progesterone. As a result, _____ stops and the _____ mucus thickens, making fertilization difficult.

60. _____ are steroid hormones synthesized from _____, and they work to stimulate or control the development and maintenance of male characteristics.

61. Giving a woman low doses of _____ increases blood estrogen levels. This action reduces _____

_____.

62. The most effective oral contraceptives contain two synthetic hormones, a _____ and _____, a synthetic progesterone. When taken consistently, this hormone combination keeps the blood levels of estrogen and progesterone high, signaling the _____ that further secretion of these hormones is not needed.

63. Androgens are primarily used in the treatment of hypogonadism, hypopituitarism, eunuchism (absence of testes or undeveloped gonads in a male), cryptorchidism (undescended testes), oligospermia (lack of sperm in the semen), and general androgen deficiency in males. The most commonly used androgen is _____.

84

Chapter **16** **Hormones and Drugs for Osteoporosis**

64. _____ are oral contraceptives that contain only progestin rather than a combination of estrogen and progestin. They increase blood levels of _____, turning off the hormone pathway with positive feedback, which prevents _____. They are not as effective as combination oral contraceptives, and most must be taken daily.

Match the name of the drug with the description of its side effects and adverse reactions. You may use the drugs more than once. Some descriptions may match more than one drug.

Descriptions

65. _____ Side effects include breast tenderness, breakthrough bleeding, fluid retention, weight gain, and acne.

66. _____ Adverse reactions may include heart attack, increased risk of blood clotting, excessive bleeding, risk of hormone-sensitive cancers, liver impairment, gallstones, and pancreatitis.

67. _____ Adverse reactions with long-term, high-dose therapy could be liver tumor, liver cancer, and hepatitis. Possible adverse effects could also include jaundice, a decreased sperm count, gynecomastia, impotence, and urinary retention.

68. _____ Adverse reactions may include blood clot formation, hypertension, liver toxicity, growth of hormone-sensitive cancers, increase of serum potassium level, and interaction with other drugs that increase potassium levels.

69. _____ Side effects include edema caused by sodium retention, acne, hirsutism, male pattern baldness, mouth irritation, diarrhea, nausea, and vomiting.

Drugs
A. Perimenopausal HRT drugs
B. Oral contraceptives
C. Androgens

TEACHING PATIENTS AND FAMILIES ABOUT SEX HORMONE REPLACEMENT AND CONTRACEPTION DRUGS

Fill in the blanks for each of the topics below regarding what is important to teach patients and families about sex hormone replacement and contraception drugs

70. Quit or reduce _____ during the time you take perimenopausal HRT and oral contraceptive drugs to reduce your risk for blood clots, heart attacks, and strokes.

71. Check the color of the roof of your mouth and the whites of your eyes weekly for the presence of a _____ tinge because perimenopausal HRT and oral contraceptive drugs can impair the _____. If you see this yellowing, report is to your healthcare provider as soon as possible.

72. Use an additional method of _____ during the first cycle because oral contraceptives require a full cycle before they are effective.

73. Take the oral contraceptive with _____ once daily, at the same time each day for best effect and to help you remember to take it. Oral contraceptives are only _____ if taken as _____.

74. Make sure your healthcare provider is aware of other prescribed drugs or over-the-counter drugs you are taking in order to avoid _____.

75. Do not increase the dose of _____ without consulting your healthcare provider if you do not see the expected effects within the first _____ months because response to the drug may take several months.

76. When taking androgen steroids, report any new or troublesome symptoms that may develop, including

_____

_____

_____

77. If you are taking androgen steroids _____ or _____, for best absorption do not eat, drink, smoke, or chew tobacco until the drug is dissolved.

78. If you are using a _____ form of the drug, do not let women or children come into contact with the areas where you have applied it to prevent them from absorbing the drug.

DRUGS FOR OSTEOPOROSIS

Match the name of the drug with the correct description of the actions, uses, side effects, and adverse reactions. You may use the names of the drugs more than once.

Descriptions

Drugs
A. Bisphosphonates
B. Estrogen agonists/ antagonists
C. Osteoclast mono- clonal antibodies

79. _____ Calcium-modifying drugs that prevent bones from losing calcium and in- crease by moving blood calcium into the bone, binding to calcium in the bone, and preventing osteoclasts from destroying bone cells and resorbing calcium. They also prevent certain white blood cells from damaging or de- stroying bone.

80. _____ Common side effects of these drugs are muscle spasms, nausea, and indiges- tion. Some people have hot flashes, sodium retention, and edema formation.

81. _____ This drug can cause allergic reactions and possible anaphylaxis. The risk increases with repeated dosage of the drug. Jaw osteonecrosis can also occur.

82. _____ Common side effects are headache, esophageal reflux, and nausea.

83. _____ Drugs that activate estrogen receptors in the bone to promote calcium reten- tion in the bone and block estrogen receptors in breast tissue and uterine tissue. These opposing responses increase bone density and prevent excessive growth of breast tissue that can lead to cancer and overgrowth of uterine endometrial tissues that can lead to excessive uterine bleeding.

84. _____ Skin rashes and muscle and joint pain are the most common side effects.

85. _____ A possible adverse effect is the increased risk for thrombotic events, which include deep vein thrombosis, stroke, myocardial infarction, and pulmonary embolism.

86. _____ Antibodies directed against immature osteoclasts. Binding of the antibodies to these cells prevents them from maturing and reducing bone density.

87. _____ Jawbone necrosis (osteonecrosis) can develop with tooth extraction or other invasive dental procedures in which the jawbone is damaged. This adverse reaction is more common in patients taking higher doses or the intravenous form of the drug.

88. _____ Additional uses are the prevention of skeletal fractures in patients with bone metastases and multiple myeloma, Paget disease, and the treatment of cancer- induced hypercalcemia.

TEACHING PATIENTS AND FAMILIES ABOUT DRUGS FOR OSTEOPOROSIS

Fill in the blanks for each of the topics below regarding what is important to teach patients and families about drugs for osteoporosis.

89. Take bisphosphonates early in the morning, right after breakfast, and _____

_____.

90. Remain in the upright position (sitting, standing, or walking) for at least _____ after taking these drugs to prevent esophageal irritation and reflux.

91. Do not _____ while taking estrogen agonists/antagonists to prevent forming dangerous blood clots that could cause a stroke or heart attack.

92. Avoid excessive _____ and _____ intake to prevent _____.

93. If you start having _____, or just don't feel right when you are receiving osteoclast monoclonal antibodies, call for help immediately.

94. Be sure to inform your dentist or oral surgeon that you are taking a _____ or receiving _____

_____ before you have any tooth extraction or invasive dental procedure involving the jawbone.

PRACTICE QUIZ

1. Bone density requires a constant supply of calcium. What supplement does dietary calcium need in order to be absorbed in the intestinal tract?
   a. Vitamin C
   b. Milk
   c. Estrogen
   d. Activated Vitamin D

2. Given that strengths and types are varied for different brands of hormones, which hormone when prescribed cannot be exchanged for another brand?
   a. Adrenal hormones
   b. Thyroid hormone agonists and antithyroid hormones
   c. Perimenopausal HRT drugs and oral contraceptives
   d. Estrogen agonists/antagonists

3. Hypothyroidism can occur in children, even from birth. How long must a child with this disorder take thyroid hormone replacement drugs?
   a. Until the child reaches puberty
   b. At least 2 years
   c. For entire life
   d. Until the child reaches 18 years old

4. Thyroid hormone agonists are safe and necessary to use during pregnancy to protect the fetus. When can mothers being treated with thyroid hormone agonists NOT use this drug?
   a. During breast-feeding
   b. While taking oral contraceptives
   c. 1 month before delivery
   d. 2 months after delivery

5. Adults over 65 years are usually prescribed a lower initial dose of thyroid hormone agonists because they are more likely to have what effects?
   a. Nausea, dizziness, and vomiting
   b. Cushing disease
   c. Blood clotting and edema
   d. Serious adverse cardiac and nervous system effects

6. How long must thyroid-suppressing drugs be taken before the patient starts to see an effect?
   a. 1 year
   b. 3 to 4 weeks
   c. 6 months
   d. 1 week

7. Which class of drugs cannot be taken during pregnancy or breast-feeding?
   a. Thyroid hormone agonists
   b. Estrogen agonists/antagonists
   c. Antithyroid drugs
   d. Warfarin

8. For which patients are the drugs used to suppress adrenal hormone production NOT approved?
   a. Patients over 65
   b. Patients under the age of 2
   c. Male patients
   d. Women who are pregnant or breast-feeding

9. The symptoms of menopause are caused by low levels of estrogen and high levels of what hormone?
   a. Follicle stimulating hormone (FSH)
   b. Gonadotropin-releasing hormone (GnRH)
   c. Luteinizing hormone (LH)
   d. Progesterone

10. Which one of the following is NOT a symptom of hypothyroidism?
    a. Body temperature below normal
    b. Constipation
    c. Increased facial and body hair, decreased scalp hair
    d. Weight loss

11. What is the most common cause of hyperthyroidism?
    a. Goiter
    b. Basedow disease
    c. Grave disease
    d. Pretibial myxedema

12. What are the names of the two layers of the adrenal gland?
    a. Cortex and medulla
    b. Capsule and medulla
    c. Adrenal fat and the kidney
    d. Zona glomerulosa and zona reticularis

13. Mifepristone is only approved for patients with hypercortisolism and what other disease?
    a. Hyperaldosteronism
    b. Type 2 diabetes
    c. Menstrual irregularities
    d. Hypoglycemia

14. What causes the hot flashes (hot flushes) with facial redness and feelings of overheating during menopause?
    a. The secretion of gonadotropin-releasing hormone (GnRH) in the brain
    b. The luteinizing hormone causing the ovary to secrete progesterone
    c. High levels of FSH acting on blood vessels to make them dilate suddenly
    d. Ovulation

15. What is the process that causes old bone cells to be continually removed from bones?
    a. Osteoblastic
    b. Osteoclastic
    c. Osteoporosis
    d. Menopause

17 Drug Therapy for Diabetes

TYPES OF DIABETES MELLITUS

For each of the statements below, indicate whether it describes diabetes mellitus type 1 (1), diabetes mellitus type 2 (2), or both types 1 and 2 (B).

1. _____ Autoimmune disorder

2. _____ The pancreas continues to make some insulin.

3. _____ Beta cells of pancreas that manage insulin have been destroyed.

4. _____ Long-term complications can shorten the life span of the individual.

5. _____ May not have to take insulin if controlled adequately

6. _____ Body's immune system creates antibodies against insulin-secreting cells in the pancreas.

7. _____ Usually caused by genetic predisposition or exposure to certain viruses

8. _____ There is a reduced response to insulin, known as insulin resistance.

9. _____ Frequently diagnosed in childhood

10. _____ Frequently caused by obesity and decreased physical activity

11. _____ The pancreas produces no insulin.

12. _____ The patient must take insulin for the remainder of his or her life unless receiving a pancreas transplant.

MATCHING

Match the drugs listed in the left column with the drug categories on the right.

Drugs

13. _____ Dulaglutide

14. _____ Canagliflozin

15. _____ NovoLog

16. _____ Humulin R

17. _____ Metformin

18. _____ Pioglitazone

19. _____ Glimepiride

20. _____ Saxagliptin

21. _____ Levemir

22. _____ Alogliptin

23. _____ Acarbose

24. _____ Second-generation sulfonylurea agents

25. _____ Empagliflozin

26. _____ Lixisenatide

27. _____ Pramlintide

Drug Categories

A. Insulin stimulators (secretogogues)
B. Biguanides
C. Insulin sensitizers
D. Alpha-glucosidase inhibitors
E. Incretin mimetics
F. Amylin analogs
G. DPP-4 inhibitors
H. Sodium-glucose cotransport inhibitors
I. Insulin

KEY TERMS

Match the term with the correct definition.

Definition

28. _____ is a condition of higher-than-normal blood glucose levels.

29. _____ is a protein hormone produced by the pancreas or injected as a drug that binds to insulin receptors on many cells, which then promotes the movement of glucose from the blood into the cells.

30. _____ is a condition of lower-than-normal blood glucose levels.

31. _____ is a common chronic endocrine problem in which either the lack of insulin or poor function of insulin impairs glucose metabolism and leads to problems in fat and protein metabolism.

32. _____ is a category of noninsulin antidiabetic drug that lowers blood glucose levels by preventing the kidney from reabsorbing glucose that was filtered from the blood into the urine. This glucose then remains in the urine and is excreted rather than moved back into the blood.

33. _____ are oral and injectable drugs that use a variety of mechanisms other than binding to insulin receptors to help lower blood glucose levels back to the normal range.

34. _____ is a category of noninsulin antidiabetic drugs that help prevent hyperglycemia by reducing the amount of the DPP-4, which inactivates the normal incretins, GLP and GIP. This allows the naturally produced incretins to be present and work with insulin to control blood glucose levels.

35. _____ is an oral noninsulin antidiabetic drug that lowers blood glucose levels by preventing enzymes in the intestinal tract from breaking down starches and more complex sugars into glucose.

36. _____ is an injectable noninsulin antidiabetic drug similar to natural amylin, which is a hormone produced by pancreatic beta cells and is co-secreted with insulin in response to blood glucose elevation. It prevents hyperglycemia by delaying gastric emptying and making the patient feel full.

37. _____ is a category of noninsulin antidiabetic drug that acts like the natural gut hormones (e.g., GLP-1) that are secreted in response to food in the stomach. They work with insulin to prevent blood glucose levels from becoming too high after meals by slowing the rate of gastric emptying.

38. _____ is a sugar-based nutrient critically important for energy production in cells and organs.

39. _____ is an oral noninsulin antidiabetic drug that lowers blood glucose levels by reducing the glucose the liver releases and by reducing how much and how fast the intestines absorb the glucose in food.

40. _____ is a category of oral noninsulin antidiabetic drugs that lowers blood glucose levels by making insulin receptors more sensitive to insulin, which increases cellular uptake and use of glucose.

41. _____ is a category of oral noninsulin antidiabetic drugs that lowers blood glucose levels by triggering the release of insulin stored in the beta cells of the pancreas. The sulfonylureas and the meglitinides are the two classes of drugs in this category.

Term

A. Alpha-glucosidase inhibitors
B. Amylin analogs
C. Biguanides
D. Diabetes mellitus
E. DPP-4 inhibitors
F. Glucose
G. Hyperglycemia
H. Hypoglycemia
I. Incretin mimetics
J. Insulin
K. Insulin sensitizers
L. Insulin stimulators
M. Noninsulin antidiabetic drugs
N. Sodium-glucose cotransport inhibitors

90

SIDE AND ADVERSE EFFECTS OF DRUGS FOR DIABETES

42. Complete the table.

CATEGORIES	SIDE EFFECTS	ADVERSE EFFECTS
Insulin Stimulators	_____ _____ _____ _____ _____	Hypoglycemia Can cause the beta cells of the pancreas to stop producing insulin, a condition known as "secondary beta cell failure." Can affect the liver and increase liver enzyme levels.
Biguanides	Nausea Diarrhea Flatulence Weight loss	_____ _____ _____ _____ _____
Insulin Sensitizers	Hypoglycemia Headache Sneezing Sore throat	_____ _____ _____ _____
Alpha-Glucosidase Inhibitors	_____ _____ _____ _____ _____	Inflammation of the bowel such as colitis Crohn disease or intestinal obstruction Hypoglycemia Liver impairment with elevated liver enzyme levels.
Incretin Mimetics	Nausea, vomiting Diarrhea Upper respiratory tract symptoms Weight loss	_____ _____ _____ _____
_____	Nausea Vomiting Headache Abdominal pain Weight loss and fatigue Dizziness	Severe hypoglycemia Pancreatitis

Continued

Chapter **17** **Drug Therapy for Diabetes**

CATEGORIES	SIDE EFFECTS	ADVERSE EFFECTS
DPP-4 Inhibitors	_____ _____ _____ _____ _____ _____ _____ _____ _____	Hypoglycemia Allergic reactions with symptoms of hives, facial swelling, and itching Acute and even fatal pancreatitis Severe arthralgia (joint pain) Bullous pemphigoid, a rare skin condition that results in large, fluid-filled blisters that most often occur in the lower abdomen, upper thighs, or armpits
Sodium-Glucose Cotransport Inhibitors	Increased need to urinate Patients using glucose strips to check for glucose in the urine will see a positive result most of the time because glucose is excreted in the urine. Weight loss initially through the loss of fluid followed by loss of fat mass	_____ _____ _____ _____ _____ _____ _____ _____
_____	Mild allergic reactions such as swelling, itching, or redness around the injection site, and changes to the skin at injection sites	Hypoglycemia leading to loss of consciousness, and even death. Injection site infections

MULTIPLE CHOICE

For each of the drug categories listed below, check all items that describe what should be taught to patients and families.

43. Insulin stimulators (secretogogues)

   a. _____ Take these drugs at least 2 hours before meals.

   b. _____ Hypoglycemia symptoms include hunger pangs, nervousness, confusion, and tremors.

   c. _____ Check with healthcare provider before taking any over-the-counter or prescription drugs to ensure stabilized blood glucose levels.

   d. _____ Avoid exercise at least 4 hours after taking these drugs.

44. Biguanides

   a. _____ Avoid drinking alcohol as this increases chance of developing lactic acidosis.

   b. _____ Common side effects include rashes, increased urine output, and headaches.

   c. _____ Check with healthcare provider about stopping and starting drug if radiopaque dye is being used.

   d. _____ Laboratory tests are important due to risk of cardiovascular disease and B_{12} deficiency.

45. Insulin sensitizers

    a. _____ If you miss a dose, take as soon as possible and do not double dosages.

    b. _____ Report any of the following to your healthcare provider: itching, hives, swelling, changes in vision, swelling of feet or angles, rapid weight gain, or symptoms of hyperglycemia.

    c. _____ Avoid alcohol, which can affect blood glucose levels.

    d. _____ Avoid all foods with sugar if symptoms of hypoglycemia are present.

    e. _____ Check your blood sugar on a monthly basis.

46. Alpha-glucosidase inhibitors

    a. _____ When taking these drugs, you should avoid all exercise.

    b. _____ These drugs must be taken at the end of meals to get the most benefit.

    c. _____ The drug's effect on blood sugar levels following meals depends on the amount of protein in the meal.

    d. _____ Avoid alcohol while taking these drugs as they increase risk of liver impairment.

47. Incretin mimetics

    a. _____ If you have difficulty breathing, a "lump" in your throat, or swelling of the mouth and tongue, call 911.

    b. _____ Alcohol increases the risk of pancreatic inflammation.

    c. _____ If a dose is missed, double your next dosage.

    d. _____ Give subcutaneous injection in thigh, upper arm, or abdomen.

    e. _____ Inject the drug 60 minutes *after* meals.

48. Amylin analogs

    a. _____ Opened vials and injectable pens should be refrigerated or used within 28 days.

    b. _____ The drug should warm to room temperature before injecting.

    c. _____ Give this drug right after your meal.

    d. _____ Do not mix pramlintide with insulin in the same syringe.

    e. _____ Dispose all used syringes and needles in a plastic bag.

    f. _____ Do not drive or operate machinery until you know whether this drug causes dizziness.

49. DPP-4 inhibitors

    a. _____ If a dose is accidentally missed, do not double up on the subsequent drug dose.

    b. _____ Report any hypoglycemia incidents to your healthcare provider.

    c. _____ Report symptoms of allergic reaction, angioedema, or pancreatitis to your healthcare provider.

    d. _____ These drugs are safe to use if you are pregnant or breast-feeding.

50. Sodium-glucose cotransport inhibitors

    a. _____ Check your blood sugar at regular intervals.

    b. _____ Report any weight gain to your healthcare provider.

    c. _____ Report signs of UTI or vaginal infection.

    d. _____ Limit fluids throughout the day.

    e. _____ Glucose will be present in your urine while taking this drug.

93

51. Insulin

    a. _____ When symptoms of hypoglycemia are present, avoid eating or drinking anything until the symptoms pass.

    b. _____ When symptoms of hyperglycemia are present, eat or drink something containing sugar.

    c. _____ Seek emergency treatment for symptoms of ketoacidosis.

    d. _____ Keep appointments with your healthcare provider to test your blood glucose levels.

    e. _____ Insulin vial must be stored at room temperature.

    f. _____ Shake insulin vial vigorously before drawing the insulin up.

    g. _____ Avoid alcohol because it can intensify hypoglycemia.

    h. _____ Carry a readily available source of protein at all times, in case you develop symptoms of hypoglycemia.

PRACTICE QUIZ

1. What is the purpose of glucose, a sugar-based nutrient?
   a. Binds insulin receptors on many cells
   b. Metabolizes within the cells to generate the body's energy
   c. Prevents hyperglycemia
   d. Is released within the body when energy is low

2. How does insulin, a protein hormone produced by the pancreas, prevent hyperglycemia?
   a. Provides the muscles with energy
   b. Prevents the body from storing sugar
   c. Prevents the kidney from eliminating glucose
   d. Allows body cells to take up, use, and store carbohydrate, fat, and protein

3. How does glucagon work to prevent low blood glucose levels?
   a. Triggers the release of glucose from the liver and skeletal muscle when blood glucose is lower than normal
   b. Prevents the release of insulin from the pancreas when blood glucose is lower than normal
   c. Protects cells from releasing too much energy when blood glucose is lower than normal
   d. Ensures sufficient insulin is released from the pancreas when blood glucose is lower than normal

4. Why do the neurons and the brain require a continuous supply of glucose from the blood?
   a. The brain and neurons are continuously working to keep the body functioning.
   b. The brain stores only a minimal amount of fat, which must be continuously replenished.
   c. The brain is unable to store any glucose.
   d. The brain and neurons use significantly more glucose than other parts of the body.

5. What is the primary cause of diabetes mellitus?
   a. An overproduction of insulin that inhibits glucose from functioning adequately.
   b. Glucose is not released in adequate amounts into the blood stream.
   c. The brain and neurons do not receive an adequate supply of glucose, and therefore the organs do not operate efficiently.
   d. Glucose movement from the blood into cells and organs is impaired.

6. What are some of the complications of uncontrolled or poorly controlled diabetes mellitus?
   a. Sterility
   b. Restrictions in activities
   c. Reduced functions of all organs and tissues
   d. Blood pressure lower than normal

7. What causes the potentially fatal condition known as ketoacidosis?
   a. A patient with diabetes mellitus eats an excess of protein.
   b. The body uses stored fat for energy in place of glucose.
   c. The pancreas creates an excess of insulin, causing the body to use muscle protein for energy in place of glucose.
   d. A patient with diabetes mellitus drinks an excess of alcohol.

8. While type 1 diabetes onset is sudden and severe and quickly diagnosed, why is type 2 diabetes usually not diagnosed as quickly?
   a. Type 2 diabetes is only diagnosed if blood glucose levels are tested regularly.
   b. In type 2 diabetes, the pancreas still produces some insulin, so symptoms may not occur until complications begin.
   c. In some individuals, type 2 diabetes symptoms may eventually dissipate over time.
   d. Type 2 diabetes often presents as pancreatitis, and the other symptoms are overlooked.

9. When a patient is first diagnosed with type 2 diabetes, what is the best first line of treatment for the chronic disease?
    a. Insulin injections to replace the levels no longer produced by the pancreas
    b. Noninsulin antidiabetic drugs to control blood glucose levels
    c. No treatment is recommended until consistent testing of blood glucose levels indicates a consistent higher-than-normal level.
    d. Patient should try diet and exercise first to determine whether those measures will help maintain a target blood glucose level.

10. What is necessary for insulin stimulator oral drugs to lower blood glucose levels?
    a. The patient must take the drug consistently on a daily basis to ensure effectiveness.
    b. The patient must have some functioning beta cells within the pancreas.
    c. The patient must have a blood glucose level that is closer to normal range.
    d. The patient must maintain a healthy diet and program of exercise.

11. What is the only drug available in the biguanides category of drugs?
    a. Metformin
    b. Miglitol
    c. Exenatide
    d. Saxagliptin

12. Which category of drug is most often recommended for patients who have high blood sugar following meals?
    a. Insulin sensitizers
    b. Alpha-glucosidase inhibitors
    c. Incretin mimetics
    d. Amylin analogs

13. Where should subcutaneous injections be given?
    a. Rotate between upper arm and upper thigh.
    b. Rotate between both sides of lower abdomen.
    c. Select upper arm, upper thigh, or abdomen and consistently use the same location.
    d. Rotate among upper arm, upper thigh, and abdomen.

14. What is considered a normal fasting blood glucose level?
    a. 70–90 ml/dL
    b. 60–100 ml/dL
    c. 75–115 ml/dL
    d. 80–90 ml/dL

15. Why should insulin be given by the parenteral route?
    a. Because insulin must be refrigerated, it can upset the stomach.
    b. It is necessary to use a faster route of administration for insulin.
    c. Because insulin is destroyed by stomach acids and intestinal enzymes
    d. To prevent stress on the pancreas

EAR AND EYE STRUCTURE AND FUNCTION TERMINOLOGY

Complete the following puzzle

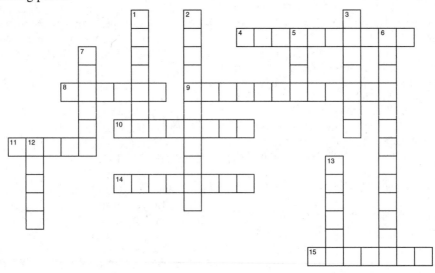

ACROSS

4. Carries messages from the special cells in the retina to the brain where we then "see" the images
8. Stirrups
9. The watery fluid that fills the space between the cornea and the lens
10. Three small bones in the middle ear.
11. The external ear
14. The S-shaped tube leading from the pinna to the ear drum
15. Tympanic membrane

DOWN

1. Hammer
2. Normal circulation of the watery fluid maintains a normal _____ pressure (IOP)
3. Ear wax
5. Muscular ring around the eye
6. Jelly-like substance that fills the posterior segment of the eye
7. Lining of the back of the eye
12. Anvil
13. Clear covering of the eye that allows light to enter

KEY TERMS

Match terms to the correct description.

Descriptions

16. _____ Liquid or ointment drugs prepared to place on the eye or the conjunctiva

17. _____ Drugs that bind to specific prostaglandin receptor sites in the eye, causing an increased outflow of aqueous humor

18. _____ Drugs that bind to receptor sites in the eye and reduce the amount of aqueous humor produced

19. _____ A type of diuretic that can also lower intraocular pressure by decreasing production of aqueous humor by 50–60%

20. _____ Drugs that increase the availability of acetylcholine to activate specific receptors, which leads to decreased production of aqueous humor and improving outflow of aqueous humor to decrease intraocular pressure

21. _____ Drugs that soften earwax

22. _____ Drugs that inhibit adrenergic receptor sites in the eye and decrease production of aqueous humor

23. _____ Drugs prepared for delivery into the external ear canal

Terms

A. Alpha-adrenergic agonists
B. Beta-adrenergic blocking agents
C. Carbonic anhydrase inhibitors (CAIs)
D. Cerumenolytics
E. Cholinergic agents
F. Ophthalmic drugs
G. Otic drugs
H. Prostaglandin agonists

EAR PROBLEMS

24. The most common ear problems that occur in the external ear and in the middle ear are _____ and

_____.

25. When these problems occur in the middle ear, _____ and _____ are given systemically, most often by the oral route.

26. When these common ear problems occur in the pinna and the ear canal, they are most often managed by

_____ drug application.

27. Drugs that are prepared to apply into the external ear canal are _____ drugs.

28. The length and angle of ear canals differ between young children and adults. In adults, the ear canal tilts downward, is longer, and is slightly curved in an S-shape. In children, the canal is shorter and straighter. These differences require distinct techniques when instilling otic drugs.

Adults: _____

_____

Children: _____

_____

29. What symptoms may occur with excessive wax build up in the ear?

_____

_____

30. Name the type of drugs that soften earwax and can be instilled before irrigation.

_____

31. Never place a drug into the ear canal or irrigate the ear canal if there is _____ present because it could enter the middle ear and cause an infection. Also, do not place drugs into the ear canal if the patient is dizzy, as dizziness will be increased.

32. Number in correct order the steps for instilling topical drugs into the patient's ear canal.
    ☐ Wash hands and don a pair of clean gloves.
    ☐ Remind the patient to keep the head in this position for 2–3 minutes to allow the drops to flow.
    ☐ Read the label of the drug carefully to ensure that it is for "otic" use. Never put any solution in the ear that is not labeled specifically for use in ears.
    ☐ Warm the ear drops to room temperature.
    ☐ For an older child or adult, pull the pinna up and back.
    ☐ Using the applicator, place only the prescribed number of drops into the patient's ear. Aim the drops onto the side of the ear canal and let them run into the ear.
    ☐ Remove your gloves and wash hands.
    ☐ Make sure that the patient's eardrum is intact. This may require assessment by the RN or other healthcare provider. Never give an ear drug if there is damage to the eardrum.
    ☐ Insert a cotton ball into the opening of the ear canal to keep the drops from rolling out of the ear.
    ☐ For a young child (younger than 3), gently pull the pinna down and back.
    ☐ Ask the patient to lie down with the head turned so that the affected ear is turned upward; if the patient sitting in a chair, tilt the patient's head so the affected ear is up
    ☐ Verify the drug using the nine rights of drug administration.

EYE PROBLEMS

33. Problems that affect the eyes and vision that can be managed with drug therapy are _____,

    _____, and _____.

34. Drugs for these problems are _____ drugs, which come in liquid drops or ointment form to place on the eye or the conjunctiva.

35. Pupil constriction is _____. Pupil dilation is _____.

36. Most _____ and _____ drugs used to treat eye problems have an ophthalmic form that can be given topically.

37. Number in order the steps for giving eye drops or ointments to a patient.
    ☐ Without pressing on the eyelid, gently blot or wipe away any excess drug or tears with a tissue.
    ☐ Wash your hands and put on gloves.
    ☐ Wash your hands again.
    ☐ Replace contact lenses as appropriate.
    ☐ Remove your gloves.
    ☐ Remind the patient that his or her vision will be blurry and not to drive until the vision clears.
    ☐ Recap the tube or bottle.
    ☐ Make sure the patient is not wearing contact lenses; if needed, ask the patient to remove them.
    ☐ If both eyes are to receive the same drug and one eye is infected, use two separate bottles or tubes and carefully label each with "right" or "left" for the correct eye.
    ☐ Hold the eye-drop bottle or ointment tube (with the cap off) like a pencil, with the tip pointing down.
    ☐ Have the patient sit in a chair while you stand behind the patient (or alternatively stand in front of the patient who is sitting in a chair or over the patient who is lying in bed).
    ☐ Gently release the lower lid.
    ☐ Gently pull the lower lid down against the patient's cheek, forming a small pocket.

- ☐ For ointment, squeeze a small amount out onto a tissue (without touching the tip to the tissue) and discard this ointment.
- ☐ For eye drops, with a gloved finger gently press and hold the corner of the eye nearest the nose to close off the tear duct and prevent the drug from being absorbed systemically.
- ☐ For eye drops, gently squeeze the bottle and release the prescribed number of drops into the pocket that you have made with the patient's lower eyelid. Do not touch any part of the eye or lid with the tip of the bottle. For ointment, gently squeeze the tube and release a small amount of ointment into the pocket that you have made with the patient's lower eyelid. Do not touch any part of the eye or lid with the tip of the tube.
- ☐ Explain the procedure to the patient.
- ☐ Check to see whether only one eye is to have the drug or if both eyes are to receive the drug.
- ☐ Check the name, strength, expiration date, color, and clarity of the eye drops to be instilled. If the drug is an ointment, be sure that it is an ophthalmic (eye) preparation and not a general topical ointment.
- ☐ Ask the patient to tilt his or her head backward, with the back of the head resting against you (or the back of the chair) and look up at the ceiling.
- ☐ Ask the patient to close his or her eye gently, without squeezing the lids tightly, and roll the eye under the lid to spread the drug across the eye for about 2 minutes.

GLAUCOMA

38. Glaucoma is a chronic eye disease of increased _____ pressure that causes damage to the optic nerve.

39. If untreated, glaucoma causes loss of _____ and even blindness.

40. Glaucoma is an eye disorder resulting from too much _____.

41. Name the most common type of glaucoma.

    _____ (POAG)

42. Drug therapy for patients with glaucoma involves _____the amount of aqueous humor produced by the ciliary body or improving drainage and reabsorption of the aqueous humor. This decreases fluid pressure in

    the eye and relieves pressure on the _____ and the _____.

Match the glaucoma drugs with the corresponding action, uses, side effects, and possible adverse reactions. Each drug will be used more than once.

Corresponding Actions

43 _____ Systemic absorption may cause adverse reactions such as changes in blood pressure, and abnormal heart rhythms. Other adverse effects include double vision and retinal detachment.

44. _____ Related to sulfonamide drugs and may cause an allergic reaction in patients allergic to any sulfa drug. Oral or IV administration can cause confusion, dizziness, numbness of the hands and feet (even paralysis), severe skin infections, severe electrolyte imbalances, and liver failure.

45. _____ Help control glaucoma by binding to receptor sites in the eye and relax eye blood vessel smooth muscles, which allows these blood vessels to dilate and absorb aqueous humor

46. _____ Expected side effects of this class of drugs include tearing, stinging, redness of the eye, blurred vision, and mitosis. Systemic side effects are possible and include headache, increased saliva, increased urination, and sweating.

47. _____ Adverse effects may be bradycardia or tachycardia and a drop in blood pressure. Also, there may be allergic reaction, fatigue, and respiratory symptoms.

48. _____ If absorbed systemically, this class of drug can develop decreased heart rate, decreased blood pressure, and even heart failure. Systemic absorption can also cause bronchoconstriction and asthma symptoms.

49. _____ Can rarely experience infection, asthma, and corneal erosion (damage to the cornea)

50. _____ Class of drug that acts to reduce the amount of aqueous humor produced in the eye. In addition, these drugs improve the flow of aqueous humor out of the anterior chamber of the eye.

51. _____ Cause eye itching and eye redness when first applied. Patients can have a foreign body sensation. The iris color may change to brown, lashes may thicken and lengthen, and dark skin may appear under the eye.

52. _____ Tearing, redness, blurring of vision, burning, stinging, or sensation of foreign object are common side effects after giving the eye drops

53. _____ Decrease IOP by reducing the amount of aqueous humor produced and improving its flow. By increasing the amount of this drug, the pupil becomes smaller (miosis). This in turn increases the amount of space between the lens and the iris, allowing the aqueous fluid to flow freely decreasing IOP.

54. _____ Side effects include temporary blurring of vision, slight burning or stinging, and tearing of the eye. Later, the patient may notice less tear production and dry, itchy, or red eyes. Pupils will not dilate as easily when entering a dark room.

55. _____ Reduce the amount of aqueous humor produced from the ciliary body of the eye

56. _____ Lower IOP by reducing aqueous humor in the anterior chamber of the eye. This class of drugs is a type of diuretic.

57. _____ Slight burning or stinging with administration. Some patients may experience a bitter or sour taste in the mouth. In rare cases, redness of the conjunctiva can occur.

Drugs

A. Alpha-adrenergic agonists
B. Beta-adrenergic blocking agents
C. Anhydrase inhibitors (CAIs)
D. Cholinergic agents
E. Prostaglandin agonists

100

58. Why is it not advisable to use higher-than-prescribed doses of prostaglandin agonist?

    _____

59. When using prostaglandin agonists, if you have lighter colored eyes, what three things can change over time?

    a. _____ b._____

    c. _____

60. If you have glaucoma only in one eye, prostaglandin agonist drops should be placed in both eyes so the colors will

    match. True or False? _____

61. Do not increase the dose of beta-adrenergic antagonists or use the drug more often because excessive use increases

    the risk for _____

    _____

62. When using beta-adrenergic antagonists or cholinergic drugs, why should good lighting always be used?

    _____

    _____

63. If you have diabetes, check your blood glucose more often because beta-adrenergic antagonists can

    _____ of hypoglycemia if the drug is absorbed systemically.

64. When giving beta-adrenergic antagonists to older patients, make sure they are not taking any

    _____ drugs for a cardiac condition. If so, notify the healthcare provider. Older adults are
    more likely to have cardiac and respiratory problems from systemic absorption of eye drops.

65. Make sure to read packaging carefully as some alpha-adrenergic drugs may need to be stored in the

    _____ and _____ to maintain potency.

66. If being treated with alpha-adrenergic drugs, wear dark glasses when you are in the sunlight or other bright light

    conditions because your pupil will be _____ and your eye will be sensitive to the light.

67. If you have been prescribed to use alpha-adrenergic drugs for a limited time such as 1 week, do not continue the
    drug beyond that time period. Explain why this is true.

    _____

68. Give the main reason for immediately wiping up any spills of cholinergic drops from the patient's skin. _____

    _____

69. What two symptoms indicate a toxic level of cholinergic drugs and should be reported to a healthcare provider
    immediately?

    a. _____

    b. _____

70. Do not give carbonic anhydrase inhibitors (CAIs) to _____ and avoid during _____

    and _____.

71. After giving eye drops, ask the patient to close his or her eyes for _____. This reduces the amount of drug
    absorbed systemically. A second option to reduce systemic absorption of the drug is to apply gentle pressure with

    the index finger over the _____ for about 3 minutes after giving the eye drops.

1. Cerumenolytic drugs are sold over-the-counter and usually contain what chemical?
   a. Apraclonidine
   b. Brinzolamide
   c. Carbamide peroxide
   d. Carbastat

2. Aqueous humor is produced by which part of the eye?
   a. Retina
   b. Ciliary body
   c. Optic nerve
   d. Lacrimal gland

3. What is the normal intraocular pressure of the eye?
   a. 10 to 20 mm Hg
   b. 30 to 40 mm Hg
   c. 32 psi
   d. 120/80 to 140/90

4. Which institute provides an excellent Internet resource for healthcare professionals, patients, and families about various eye disorders, with information and photographs?
   a. The John Hopkins Wilmer Eye Institute (http://www.hopkinsmedicine.org/wilmer)
   b. The National Eye Institute (NEI) (https://nei.nih.gov/)
   c. The Vanderbilt Eye Institute (https://www.vanderbilthealth.com/eyeinstitute/)
   d. Rand Eye Institute (https://www.randeye.com/about-us/)

5. Why is glaucoma called a "thief-in-the-night" disease?
   a. Patient typically has no symptoms other than a gradual loss of peripheral side vision.
   b. Patient often has night blindness as a first symptom.
   c. Patient has sudden loss of vision.
   d. Patient only experiences symptoms when first waking up in the morning.

6. What is the rare type of glaucoma that causes a sudden increase of intraocular pressure and patient experiences severe headache, nausea and vomiting, and halo-effect around lights?
   a. Primary open angle
   b. Secondary closed angle
   c. Acute open angle
   d. Acute angle closure

7. Under what circumstances should you never instill prostaglandin agonists in a patient's eye?
   a. Headaches and sinus congestion
   b. Scratches or infection
   c. Dark coloring under the eye
   d. Dilated pupil

8. What suffix (word ending) do beta-blockers have?
   a. "ine"
   b. "mide"
   c. "olol"
   d. "mic"

9. Patients with glaucoma may have unequal size of what part of the eye? If this situation exists, you should consult with patient's healthcare provider.
   a. Iris
   b. Eyelid
   c. Retina
   d. Pupil

10. What sudden changes related to cholinergic drugs should be reported to a healthcare provider immediately?
    a. Nausea and vomiting
    b. Increased blood pressure and heart rate, and difficulty breathing
    c. Anxiety
    d. Iris color changes to brown

11. Carbonic anhydrase inhibitors should not be given to patients with what condition?
    a. Sulfa allergy
    b. Diabetes
    c. Glaucoma
    d. Food allergies

12. Though rare, what side effects are possible with cerumenolytics?
    a. Loss of hearing for 2–3 minutes
    b. Popping sounds in the ear
    c. Redness, itching, or rash
    d. Burning sensation in the ear canal

13. What patient action will provide maximum effectiveness of treatment when given cerumenolytics?
    a. A warm, moist cloth placed over the ear
    b. Heating the drops before giving
    c. Cooling the drops before giving
    d. Remaining lying down for 5 minutes for optimum absorption

14. What should a patient be taught to do if there is a sudden decrease or loss of vision during ophthalmic drug therapy?
    a. Remain lying down until vision returns.
    b. Rinse eyes with water or saline solution.
    c. Call 911 or go to the nearest emergency room.
    d. Contact the healthcare provider.

15. What is the usual time period of drug therapy for glaucoma?
    a. 2 to 6 months
    b. The rest of the patient's life
    c. 3 weeks
    d. Until peripheral vision is restored

19 Over-the-counter Drugs, Herbal and Alternative Drugs, and Vitamins and Minerals

OVER-THE-COUNTER DRUGS (OTC)

True or False

Indicate whether each of the following statements is True (T) or False (F).

1. _____ Instruct the patient to always read the instructions and possible side effects for taking OTC drugs on a reputable Internet source.

2. _____ OTC drugs and supplements, as opposed to prescription drugs, are safer and can be taken in higher doses and for longer periods of time than the instructions suggest.

3. _____ There are no adverse interactions between OTC drugs and other drugs, food, alcohol, or other medical conditions the patient has because they are created to treat specific symptoms.

4. _____ A pharmacist can be consulted if the patient is unsure about side effects of OTC drugs.

5. _____ Responses to the drug vary from person to person.

6. _____ The patient should be informed that it is more cost-effective and safer to buy OTC drugs online.

7. _____ To avoid poisoning, a parent should give children one-half the adult dose.

8. _____ Always follow the age limits listed. If the label says the product should not be given to a child younger than 2 years, do not give it.

9. _____ Generic OTC drugs are often less expensive than brand names of the same drug.

10. _____ Drugs should be discarded if they are past the expiration date and if the packaging or instructions are missing.

11. _____ OTC drugs can be used by other family members or friends with similar symptoms because it is not a prescription written expressly for the patient.

12. _____ Giving a child a drug containing alcohol is acceptable as the child is not taking as high a dose as an adult.

13. _____ Always use the child-resistant cap and store drugs away from children.

14. _____ It is advisable to purchase OTC drugs that are multipurpose and, therefore, may treat other symptoms as well as those the patient has.

15. What is the website for educating you and your patients with current evidence-based research on various CAM

    therapies? _____

16. How do the FDA regulations differ for dietary supplements and prescription/OTC drugs?

    _____

    _____

    _____

    _____

17. If a dietary supplement is unsafe or ineffective, the FDA must prove this with scientific-based evidence. What is a supplement that was banned by the agency because it caused heart problems and other serious side effects when combined with caffeine?

    _____

18. What is the major criticism of herbal supplements?

    _____

    _____

    _____

    _____

19. What are three phytoestrogens promoted as a "natural" therapy for menopause and hormone replacement that have not been proven to be any more effective than conventional hormone therapies?

    _____   _____   _____

20. Name three herbal products that are most likely to cause dangerous interactions with any prescription drugs the patient may be taking.

    _____   _____   _____

21. Calcium derived from oyster shell can contain what three dangerous substances?

    _____   _____   _____

VITAMINS

Match the name of the vitamin with description of actions and deficiencies. Each vitamin will be used more than once.

Descriptions   **Vitamins**

22. _____ Important for vision, gene characteristics, reproduction, embryo growth   Vitamin A
and development, healthy immune system function; used to treat celiac,   Vitamin D
colitis, specific eye diseases, and night blindness   Vitamin E
                                                                              Vitamin K
23. _____ Water soluble and functions as a coenzyme in the metabolism of protein,   Vitamin B12
carbohydrates, and fat   Vitamin B9
                                                                              Vitamin B3
24. _____ Antiseizure drugs reduce the levels of this vitamin, and sulfasalazine pre- Vitamin B6
vents intestinal absorption of it.   Vitamin B2
                                                                              Vitamin B1
25. _____ Assists in formation of blood-formatting factors

26. _____ Promotes formation of collagen and healing and absorption of iron

27. _____ Helps absorption of calcium and phosphorus

28. _____ Deficiency of this vitamin causes pellagra.

29. _____ Deficiency of this vitamin causes pernicious anemia.

30. _____ Prevents damage to cell membranes

31. _____ Deficiency causes B6 anemia.

32. _____ Controls amino acid metabolism and energy release

33. _____ Synthesizes DNA and supports RBC maturation

34. _____ Deficiency causes difficulty eating and swallowing.

35. _____ Deficiency causes beriberi.

36. _____ Helps formulate red blood cells

37. _____ Controls metabolism of CHO, protein, and fats

38. _____ Deficiency can cause scurvy.

39. _____ Deficiency may cause rickets, osteomalacia, and hypoparathyroidism.

40. _____ Important for the metabolism of carbohydrates

41. _____ Deficiency causes blood-clotting disorders.

42. _____ Deficiency causes folic acid anemia.

43. Name the primary food sources for each vitamin.

Vitamin A	Vitamin D
Vitamin E	Vitamin K
Vitamin B12	Vitamin B3
Vitamin B9	Vitamin B6
Vitamin B1	Vitamin B2

Fill in the blanks

44. What are the four signs of Vitamin A overdose? _____

_____ _____ _____

45. _____ in food is destroyed if food is boiled, fried, or baked for a long time under pressure.

46. Give the alternate name for the B vitamins.

B12 _____   B9 _____

B3 _____   B6 _____

B1 _____   B2 _____

47. If niacin is taken along with some hypertension drugs, a condition called _____
may occur. Patient should be told to sit or lie down if dizziness occurs.

48. Warn patients that taking riboflavin supplements can cause urine to become _____.

49. Name the three major forms of Vitamin C.

_____ _____ _____

50. Give the therapeutic daily dose of Vitamin D supplementation for the following two conditions:

Rickets _____

Hypoparathyroidism_____

51. _____ is the antidote for warfarin (Coumadin) overdose.

MINERALS

Match the name of the mineral with the description of uses, side effects, or precautions.
Each mineral may be used more than once.

Descriptions

52. _____ Major mineral in the body and is essential for muscular and neurologic activity, especially in the cardiac system

53. _____ Part of many enzymes and is essential for normal growth and tissue repair. It functions in the mineralization of bone and in the detoxification of methanol and ethylene glycol. It plays a role in the creation of DNA and the synthesis of protein from amino acids. It is important in wound healing and functions in moving vitamin A from liver stores.

54. _____ Principal intracellular positive ion (cation) of most body tissues, acting in the maintenance of normal kidney function, contraction of muscle, and transmission of nerve impulses

55. _____ Slight deficiencies may prolong the Q-T interval and lead to a very dangerous form of ventricular tachycardia (rapid heartbeat) called torsades de pointes.

56. _____ Essential mineral for the body to make myoglobin and hemoglobin

57. _____ Electrolyte that is essential to several enzyme systems. It is important in maintaining osmotic pressure, ion balance, bone structure, muscular contraction, and nerve conduction.

58. _____ Both low and high levels of this mineral can cause fatal heart arrhythmias.

59. _____ Expected reactions to supplements of this mineral include constipation and cramping. Adverse reactions such as diarrhea, epigastric or abdominal pain may occur.

60. _____ Adverse reactions to supplements of this mineral include gastric ulceration, nausea, and vomiting. Doses in excess of 2 g produce emesis (vomiting).

Minerals

A. Calcium
B. Iron
C. Potassium
D. Magnesium
E. Zinc

Chapter **19** Over-the-counter Drugs, Herbal and Alternative Drugs, and Vitamins and Minerals

Fill in the blank.

61. _____ is essential for absorption of calcium.

62. Acute _____ intoxication produces drowsiness, lethargy, light-headedness, staggering gait, restlessness, and vomiting leading to dehydration.

63. Signs of _____ are muscle spasms; numbness and tingling of the lips and fingers; weak, brittle nails; and fractures. Symptoms of _____ are polyuria (excretion of a large amount of urine), constipation, abdominal pain, dryness of mouth, anorexia, nausea, and vomiting.

64. Fatal anaphylactic reactions can occur with _____ IV or IM administration. Hypersensitivity reactions include rash, itching, joint pain, muscle aches, and fever.

65. Describe Trousseau sign.

_____

_____

_____

66. More _____ is absorbed if taken on an empty stomach or acid environment, while taking it with meals reduces irritation and absorption by 40–50%.

67. Deficiency of _____ may cause convulsions, slowing of growth, digestive disturbances, spasticity of muscles and nerves, accelerated heartbeat, dysrhythmias, nervous conditions, and vasodilation (opening of blood vessels).

68. All _____ supplements must be diluted properly or taken with plenty of liquid to avoid producing GI ulcers.

69. Patients should be advised that taking iron supplements causes _____. Tell patients to report constipation, diarrhea, nausea, or abdominal pain to the healthcare provider.

70. List Food Sources for the following minerals:

Calcium

Zinc

Iron

Magnesium

Potassium

PRACTICE QUIZ

1. Which of the vitamins most commonly prescribed for supplementation are fat-soluble?
   a. A, C, E, and K
   b. A, D, E, and K
   c. A, B12, D, and E
   d. C, E, D, and K

2. An excess of vitamin A during pregnancy can cause birth defects in what system of the baby?
   a. Digestive system
   b. Endocrine system
   c. Central nervous system
   d. Exocrine system

3. What hidden drug is found in many cough syrups, cold drugs and mouthwash?
   a. Caffeine
   b. Sodium
   c. Magnesium
   d. Alcohol

4. Which vitamin, when given parenterally, can cause allergic reactions including feelings of warmth, pruritus, urticaria, nausea, angioedema, shortness of breath, sweating, tightness of the throat, and cyanosis?
   a. Thiamin
   b. Niacin
   c. Beta-carotene
   d. Pyridoxine

5. What kind of vitamins are readily excreted in urine and not stored in the body?
   a. Fat-soluble
   b. Botanical
   c. Water-soluble
   d. Cyclical

6. The condition of abnormally high storage levels of vitamins, which can lead to toxic symptoms, is called?
   a. Vitamin overdose
   b. Hypervitaminosis
   c. Toxic vitamin syndrome
   d. Excessive supplementation

7. Deficiency of which vitamin causes glossitis, stomatitis, diarrhea, and skin lesions?
   a. Thiamin
   b. Niacin
   c. Beta-carotene
   d. Pyridoxine

8. What condition can be caused by taking niacin with cerivastatin or red yeast rice?
   a. Rhabdomyolysis
   b. Anemia
   c. Angiomyolipoma
   d. Bartter syndrome

9. Which of the following is **NOT** a major form of vitamin C?
   a. Citric ascorbate
   b. Ascorbic acid
   c. Calcium ascorbate
   d. Sodium ascorbate

10. What is the best natural source of Vitamin D?
    a. Milk
    b. Whole grain bread
    c. Sunshine
    d. Cereals

11. If giving B1 (thiamine) to alcoholics or thiamine-deficient persons, what must be given along with the B1 in order to prevent Wernicke encephalopathy?
    a. Magnesium
    b. Saline solution
    c. Potassium
    d. Glucose

12. What over-the-counter drug should be avoided for patients with kidney and liver diseases, stomach ulcers, or bleeding disorders?
    a. Antacids
    b. Cough syrup
    c. Ibuprofen
    d. Antihistamines

109

Medication Cards

These sample medication cards have been printed on the front and back of this page so they can be easily reproduced for student use. We recommend they be photocopied double-sided and cut into 4″ by 6″ cards.

Drug Name: _____ Trade Name: _____

Major Drug Category: _____

Drug Action: _____

_____

Uses:_____

_____

Adverse Reactions: _____

_____

Drug Interactions: _____

_____

Usual Drug Dosage:_____

_____

Nursing Implications:

Assessment: _____

Diagnosis: _____

Planning: _____

Implementation: _____

Evaluation: _____

Drug Name: _____ Trade Name: _____

Major Drug Category: _____

Drug Action: _____

_____

Uses: _____

_____

Adverse Reactions: _____

_____

Drug Interactions: _____

_____

Usual Drug Dosage: _____

_____

Nursing Implications:

Assessment: _____

Diagnosis: _____

Planning: _____

Implementation: _____

Evaluation: _____

Patient ID	Diagnosis	Comments Re: Administration/Patient Response

Patient ID	Diagnosis	Comments Re: Administration/Patient Response

Medication Cards